AMAZING MEDICINE
THAT LITERALLY GROWS ON TREES!

HERE ARE JUST A FEW OF
GINKGO BILOBA'S EXCITING BENEFITS:

- Safe, permanent relief from **allergies**—over time, ginkgo biloba can dramatically reduce your sensitivity to allergens

- Real help for **Alzheimer's sufferers**—daily doses of 120 to 240 mg have led to dramatic improvement in memory loss, loss of cognitive function, loss of attention span, disorientation, and more

- An added bonus for people taking Prozac or other drugs for **depression**—ginkgo biloba can alleviate **sexual dysfunction,** one of the common side effects of antidepressant medication

- An end to **tinnitus**—victims of this annoying ringing can get real, lasting relief

- Improved blood flow throughout the body—even to the retina, where ginkgo biloba can help stop **macular degeneration**

- Relief from the breast tenderness and bloating of **PMS**—bring an end to hormone-related edema with the magic of ginkgo biloba

FEEL THE POWER OF GINKGO!

QUANTITY SALES

Most Dell books are available at special quantity discounts when purchased in bulk by corporations, organizations, or groups. Special imprints, messages, and excerpts can be produced to meet your needs. For more information, write to: Dell Publishing, 1540 Broadway, New York, NY 10036. Attention: Director, Special Markets.

INDIVIDUAL SALES

Are there any Dell books you want but cannot find in your local stores? If so, you can order them directly from us. You can get any Dell book currently in print. For a complete up-to-date listing of our books and information on how to order, write to: Dell Readers Service, Box DR, 1540 Broadway, New York, NY 10036.

GINKGO BILOBA

AN HERBAL FOUNTAIN OF YOUTH FOR YOUR BRAIN

Glenn S. Rothfeld, M.D., M.Ac., and Suzanne LeVert

An Amaranth Book

A DELL BOOK

Published by
Dell Publishing
a division of
Bantam Doubleday Dell Publishing Group, Inc.
1540 Broadway
New York, New York 10036

ISBN: 0-440-22625-2

Printed in the United States of America

Published simultaneously in Canada

December 1998

10 9 8 7 6 5 4 3 2 1

OPM

Contents

Introduction

Ginkgo Biloba:
An Ancient Tonic for Health and Longevity

Eons ago, when the first ancestors of humans noticed that chewing certain leaves seemed to give them extra energy or protect them from sickness, the field of herbal medicine was born. Through much of recorded history people looked to the plant world to provide them with medicines as well as food, shelter, and clothing. Folklore was built around the healing powers of certain herbs. Wars were fought over ownership of ginseng, a medicinal herb grown in the Orient, and over camellia sinensis (tea), an herbal beverage plentiful in the East Indies. Holy men and women revered the ginkgo biloba trees, protecting and cultivating them on the grounds of their Chinese and Japanese temples. Healers learned to prepare herbs in every manner from teas and infusions to poultices, washes, and tinctures. And no garden was complete without the beauty of healing herbs like echinacea, lavender, and feverfew.

Then came the machine age, and with it the ability to create out of chemicals what once was the province of nature. Following their successes providing Civil War soldiers with battlefield medications, pharmacists like Squibb and Eli Lilly started to produce medications and taught doctors how to use them. New drugs were more powerful, but also more risky and more expensive. Though many drugs were based on natural plant components, they usually were altered so that the potency was heightened, and the balance of natural ingredients was eliminated. Medical schools graduated generations of doctors who relied heavily on these drug therapies, and the pharmaceutical companies were constantly producing new ones. Currently, of the 200 most commonly used medications, fewer than 20 were developed before World War II.

But in the last few years, a movement has begun in medicine to turn again toward our natural world and seek answers to what it might hold. Just as a sprout of grass might grow up through a concrete sidewalk, so has herbal medicine reasserted itself in the arena of healing choices. But there is a new twist to the current use of herbal medicine (also called phytomedicine or botanical medicine). That is, the state-of-the-art science that has driven our pharmaceutical industry now analyzes the active components of herbs to standardize them, to produce them in mass quantity and in easily dispensed forms like tablets and capsules, and to hold them up to the light of clinical and experimental trials and studies.

More and more, drug companies are looking into the use of herbs either as primary medications or as sources of new ideas in drugs. Several of the larger companies have bought herbal firms or have started their own. Some herbs, like taxol and vincristine from rain forest areas of South America, have been found to have anticancer properties. Other substances, like Mexican yam and aloe, have been used in the production of new types of medications. And the search has been on for the active ingredients of herbs, so that new forms of these herbs can be produced that don't rely on the brewing of teas or the chewing of leaves.

Nowhere is this new type of herbal medicine more evident than in the exploding use of ginkgo biloba extract. Not that ginkgo itself is new. In fact, as you will read in this book, ginkgo is well over 2,500 years old. And its powerful effects on the mind and body have been known for almost as long. The ancient Chinese physicians, who explored hundreds of herbs and used them in their treatment of patients, knew of the ways that ginkgo could be used in the aiding of memory and mental clarity.

It was the growth of phytomedicine in Europe, however, that brought ginkgo biloba into prominence. Using a standardized extract form that allows the prescriber to give the exact same thing in every capsule, European researchers performed dozens of studies on the herb. Their remarkable findings are chronicled in this book. For ginkgo has potent effects on several of the major organ systems of the body.

Millions of prescriptions are given for GBE (ginkgo biloba extract) every year in Germany and other European countries. The majority of those are given to patients over the age of 60. In study after study, GBE was found to improve circulation to the brain and enhance cognitive function, memory, and clarity, just as the Chinese physicians knew centuries ago. Even Alzheimer's disease seems to be slowed in some cases by the judicious use of ginkgo. In Germany, GBE is prescribed as a medication, paid for by insurance companies, and considered a first-line treatment in the care of the geriatric population.

But one doesn't have to be elderly to derive benefits from ginkgo. Even young people have been shown to improve test scores and their ability to perform intellectual tasks when given GBE. And there seems to be a separate action on mood, so that ginkgo can have an antidepressant effect. As such, it's frequently given with another herb, St. John's wort, in the treatment of mild depression. With antidepressant medications, ginkgo seems to be helpful in modifying side effects, and can be used safely in combination with these drugs.

Ginkgo biloba also seems to have powerful effects on the immune and clotting systems of the body. It is an inhibitor of something called "platelet-aggregating factor," which plays a major role in the inflammatory process, and the stress response generally. Thus, ginkgo can be useful in many of the illnesses in which stress and inflammation are issues. In the following pages, information can be found on the usefulness of ginkgo in such varied illnesses as asthma, heart disease, and allergy.

The positive uses of ginkgo in heart disease warrant their own chapter. In clinical studies, ginkgo has been shown to improve circulation to the brain, to the heart, and to the legs. Much of the problem in atherosclerotic circulatory disease involves an abnormal clotting in the arteries, leading to blockage of the circulation. Ginkgo biloba has been shown to lessen that clotting, and to improve clinically the symptoms of poor circulation.

One of the most exciting aspects of the new style of natural medicine is its emphasis on health and on maximizing our potential, rather than merely treating a severe illness. It has been the style of modern medicine up to this point to wait until a disease process was far along, then treat the symptoms of that disease with powerful drugs. Now comes a new style, which is being called "integrative medicine" or "complementary medicine." This new field encompasses herbal medicine but also nutritional medicine (sometimes called "functional medicine"), exercise, relaxation therapies like yoga and meditation, and ancient systems of healing like acupuncture (Chinese medicine).

So taking ginkgo biloba extract might be an early step toward a healthier mind and body, but it is by no means the only step. In the following pages, we have reviewed the principles of good diet and nutrition. We have stressed the importance of exercise and staying active in the maintenance of good health. We have looked at stress and its myriad effects on the body and on the mind. And we have suggested ways of responding to the stresses of life that tend to wear us down.

Unfortunately, the same blessing that has given us the strong medications that we rely on for long, healthy life spans has cursed us with a reliance on a quick pill or capsule to solve all of our ills. Nature does not work that way, or presumably pills would be sprouting from the ground instead of whole leaves, roots, and stems. Our prehistoric ancestors had the same physiology and anatomy as we do, and while our lives are very different, it is sometimes helpful to look at their lifestyle for guidance. Paleolithic man was physically active for five to six hours per day, ate freshly found food, slept from sundown to sunup, and spent most of his time in an unstressful environment punctuated by times of acute stress (usually caused by a mastodon or other prehistoric beast bent on dinner). And he relied on the herbal plant life around him for its healing properties.

We have no mastodons to run from, but we have a constant parade of the small stresses of life: the traffic jams, squabbles, deadlines, and family angst. We eat foods from different continents in the same meal, fast foods that sit under a heat lamp all day, processed foods that didn't exist 50 years ago. We are proud of ourselves if we exercise for 20 minutes three times per week. And we toss and turn all night, or stare at the TV far into the evening. We may share physiology with our ancestors, but we share very little of their lifestyle.

However, we can share with them the use of plants and trees around us to assist in our quest for health. And at the same time, we can rely on the best modern science to ensure that those plants and trees provide us with herbs that are potent, reliable, and efficacious. Today's herbal medicine is a true blending of the ancient and the modern, of the past and the future. And ginkgo biloba, the most ancient of herbs, is appropriately leading the way toward this new vision of healing.

Glenn S. Rothfeld, M.D. M.Ac.
and Suzanne LeVert

CHAPTER 1

Ginkgo:
Where East Meets West

- Barbie, a 38-year-old publishing executive, started taking ginkgo six months ago. "I'm under constant pressure, and need to concentrate to perform my job well. Taking just one ginkgo biloba pill a day has really helped me in that area. I'm able to focus better and for longer periods of time, and am also less likely to need a cup or two (or three) of coffee to stay alert, which helps me feel better all around. I've found it to be very helpful."

- Marjorie, a 22-year-old graduate student, began taking ginkgo last year to relieve the headaches that had plagued her for years. "It was my regular doctor who recommended it," Marjorie recalls. "She was frustrated that aspirin and ibuprofen no longer helped ease the pain, and hated to see me suffer with the nausea and stomach upset these drugs caused. I can't say that I never get headaches anymore, but since I started taking ginkgo, they're fewer and farther between, and they seem to be less severe. I also feel less anxious and stressed. I don't know if that's directly because of the ginkgo or be-

cause I'm no longer plagued by these headaches,
but in any case, I'm thrilled."

- Scott Carter, a 65-year-old retired businessman,
just started taking ginkgo biloba three months ago.
"Parkinson's disease runs in my family, and I read
in a magazine that ginkgo helps keep the brain
chemicals up and running, that it may help prevent
degenerative diseases like Parkinson's from developing. I also know that doctors now use it to help
treat Alzheimer's disease. When you get to be my
age those are really things you start to worry about,
so after I talked to my doctor, I started taking it. I
hope it helps protect me from disease, but the good
news is that it's helped me already, increasing my
concentration and short-term memory. And I
haven't had a single side effect."

Barbie, Marjorie, and Scott are just three of the millions of Americans who have decided to jump on the
growing ginkgo biloba bandwagon. Some do so after
reading about the herb's properties in a magazine or a
book like this one. Others begin taking it after their
doctors or other health care practitioners recommend
it. But just what *is* ginkgo, and can it help you? Those
are the two main questions we'll answer for you in this
book.

First, it's important for you to understand that, even
though you might have heard of ginkgo only recently,
it's been used as medicine for centuries. In addition,
there have been almost 300 modern scientific studies
performed to date that verify its safety and efficacy in
treating a wide range of diseases and conditions, including:

- Asthma and allergies
- Memory loss and poor concentration
- Alzheimer's disease
- Headache
- Depression
- Heart disease
- Peripheral vascular disease
- Impotence
- Premenstrual syndrome
- Vision problems, including macular degeneration
- Tinnitus (ringing of the ears)
- Dizziness and other balance problems

How can one herb act on so many different parts of the body and alleviate so many different conditions? That's what we'll explain in more depth in Chapter 2. For now, let's take a look at where ginkgo came from and how modern medicine has begun to take note of its remarkable effects.

THE "NEW" PROMISE OF GINKGO

In October 1997, headlines in newspapers around the world proclaimed a medical breakthrough. The prestigious *Journal of the American Medical Association* had just published the remarkable results of a study on the effects of a new treatment for Alzheimer's disease, a devastating brain disorder that strikes thousands of the elderly every year. Researchers concluded that this new treatment appeared to stabilize and, in 20 percent of cases, actually improve the functioning of 309 Alzheimer's disease patients—better statistics than those for any medication yet developed. Many studies now being conducted in laboratories around the world are designed to evaluate this remarkable finding and determine just how powerful a remedy ginkgo really is. The initial results are very encouraging.

What does this new treatment consist of? Did a pharmaceutical company create a new synthetic drug? Did it employ some high-tech ingredient or method just developed?

Hardly. The substance "discovered" in 1997 to treat Alzheimer's disease is ginkgo biloba, an herb used as medicine for centuries. In fact, a story about ginkgo biloba appears in one of the first medical texts ever written, *Pen T'sao (The Great Herbal)* in 2,800 B.C., foreshadowing the twentieth-century breakthrough. According to the text, China's first emperor, Shen Nung, had a vision in which a voice whispered that the ginkgo tree standing outside his window would "restore the minds of friends and relatives." Shen Nung instructed his staff to pick some leaves and create a tea, which he then served to those people around him with memory or concentration problems. Within weeks, every one of those afflicted had regained much of their lost mental capabilities.

And so we've come full circle. As we head toward the new millennium, scientists are reaching back into the past to find more effective ways to treat human disease. They are also increasingly looking to the East, to the countries and cultures of Asia, which continue to maintain approaches to health and disease very different from our own. Asians also look to us for our remarkable technological advances in the same field. In our increasingly interdependent world, the merging of our philosophies is proving beneficial in a variety of respects, and no more so than in the area of health and medicine.

The scientific focus on ginkgo biloba and the increasing use of this herb are the latest examples of this trend. Used for centuries in China, Japan, and other Asian countries as a medicinal herb effective in the prevention and treatment of a wide variety of conditions, ginkgo biloba is now one of the most widely prescribed formulas in Europe. Doctors in Germany and France dispense more than 1.5 million prescriptions every week to patients suffering from memory loss, lack of attention, depression, circulatory disorders, and other conditions. In 1997 alone, annual sales of ginkgo surpassed $500 million in these countries, and sales are beginning to soar on this side of the Atlantic as well.

The Living Fossil

Back when dinosaurs roamed the earth, and shallow seas and murky swamps covered the continents, ginkgo biloba trees dotted the landscapes of both the Eastern and Western Hemispheres. These deciduous trees with their short branches and pale green two-lobed leaves shaped like nubby fans were as at home in the largely unpopulated Mesozoic era 200 million years ago as they are today in crowded late-twentieth-century cities. Often called the "living fossil" because of its remarkable duration—it remains the world's oldest living species of tree—it's no wonder that Steven Spielberg insisted that ginkgo trees appear in his blockbuster movie *Jurassic Park*!

Found throughout the United States today, where it is also known as the maidenhair tree, the ginkgo biloba decorates college campuses, front lawns, office complexes, and city streets. You've probably seen ginkgo trees yourself: They grow to be about 100 feet tall and are pyramidal in shape, with slender upright branches that spread wider at the top. The leaves have a distinctive shape: Each one has two lobes divided by a deep notch. The ginkgo is deciduous, which means that its leaves change color with the seasons. In the autumn, they turn a lovely buttery yellow before falling to the ground in winter.

The tree is remarkably resilient, able to withstand infection by disease, infestation by insects, and destruction by pollution and other man-made toxins. In fact, a ginkgo was the only tree to survive the 1945 atomic bomb blast in Hiroshima, and remains as part of a shrine that marks that disaster.

Indeed, it took an environmental cataclysm the magnitude of the Ice Age to threaten the ginkgo tree, almost wiping it out in North America and Europe. Ginkgo trees continued to thrive in China and Japan, however, where they were considered sacred, and where their medicinal powers were discovered and preserved. Folklore has it that ginkgo trees survived because the priests and priestesses considered them guardians of Chinese temples, and therefore blessed with strength and immortality.

For centuries, the Chinese used ginkgo not only as a tonic for the brain, but also as a remedy for asthma, bronchitis, and certain parasitic diseases. Chinese herbal texts from the fifteenth and sixteenth centuries note the use of roasted ginkgo seeds as an aid in digestion, and recommend soaking ripe ginkgo fruit in vegetable oil for 100 days before using it as a treatment for tuberculosis. Leaves were boiled to make a tea to treat diarrhea, and to make a lotion to apply to skin affected by frostbite, freckles, and sores. In Japan, herbalists discovered that the coatings of the seeds contained a powerful natural insecticide, and placed them between the pages of books or near scrolls to protect their valuable papers from insect infestation.

It wasn't until the early eighteenth century that the ginkgo tree made its way into the Western consciousness, and then only as an attractive shade tree. German physician and botanist Englebert Kaempfer was probably the first European to see the ginkgo, as he journeyed through Japan. Later, Carolus Linnaeus, the Swedish botanist who developed a system of classifying and systematizing the species of plants and animals, named the plant *ginkgo biloba* (GINKGO BILOBA: "with two lobes") because of the two-lobed shape of its leaves. The tree first arrived in Europe from China's Chekiang Province in 1727 and was planted in the city's botanical garden.

About fifty years later, in 1784, William Hamilton of Philadelphia planted the first "American" ginkgo tree in his garden (which stands in the present-day site of Woodlawn Cemetery). Gradually, the ginkgo's hearty nature and attractive appearance made it one of the most popular trees across the country. (The only drawback is its rather malodorous fruit, which has led schoolchildren to dub it the "stinkbomb tree"! But more about that later.)

Until recently, Americans have shied away from the use of botanicals—trees, shrubs, and herbs—as medicine. Certainly, they never thought of the ubiquitous ginkgo tree as a potential source of treatment for some very common and very stubborn modern ailments. Slowly but surely over the last few decades, however, we've come to appreciate the age-old tradition of botanical, or herbal, medicine.

A RETURN TO OUR ROOTS

In the last few decades, alternative therapies of all types—including herbal medicine, the Chinese tradition of acupuncture, massage therapies, and meditation—have become increasingly popular in the United States. In fact, the *New York Times* reported in October 1997 that, according to the Council for Responsible Nutrition, an estimated 100 million Americans spend about $6.5 billion a year on herbal, vitamin, and mineral supplements—more than double the $3 billion they spent in 1990. Sixty-two percent of Americans say they'll consider visiting an alternative health practitioner if conventional techniques fail them, and 84 percent of those who've sought alternative therapies say they would do so again.

Why the relatively sudden interest in other methods of healing? Simply put, Western medicine has failed us to a certain extent. Something is missing, something is out of balance with our approach. There's no doubt that we benefit from a highly sophisticated medical technology that can target and treat a specific virus or remove a tumor quite efficiently. But, although drugs and surgery may be lifesavers in certain circumstances, such as when raging bacterial infections take hold or heart attacks or accidents occur, modern medicine remains stymied by conditions of a systemic and/or chronic nature. Unfortunately, chronic diseases like allergies, heart disease, and diabetes are on the rise, and nearly 10 million American men and women will suffer one or more episodes of major depression during their lifetimes—the very conditions that a natural remedy like ginkgo can help to treat.

Within the modern Western medical tradition, physicians and researchers often divide health problems into those considered *acute* and those considered *chronic*. Acute health problems generally begin abruptly and have a single, readily identifiable cause. These conditions usually respond well and quickly to specific treatments, such as medication or surgery. When treatment succeeds in eliminating the symptoms and effects of the acute illness, doctors consider patients "cured," or brought back to a normal state of health.

Chronic conditions, on the other hand, tend to start slowly, progress slowly, and endure over several years, even over a lifetime. Sometimes doctors find it difficult to even diagnose a chronic illness, since its symptoms and course may be both subtle and unpredictable. Unlike acute disease or infection, chronic disease often has several possible, coexisting causes, ranging from genetic factors to lifestyle and environmental influences to individual physiological attributes. Almost by definition, chronic illnesses have no "cure," no simple solution.

In recent decades, many Americans have been looking to Asia for potential solutions to their chronic health problems. In general, Chinese medicine and its cousins in India and Tibet concentrate more on natural remedies, such as herbs and nutrition, and less on manmade pharmaceuticals than does Western medicine. Furthermore, and perhaps more important, these remedies are not meant simply to ease a certain symptom or "cure" a specific infection, but rather to reestablish a whole-body balance, to bring the body and the spirit back into the proper alignment and balance called health.

About a quarter of a century ago, most Americans gained their first glimpse of the remarkable tradition of Chinese medicine, of which the use of ginkgo biloba is just the latest example. In 1972, President Richard Nixon made the first official U.S. government trip in nearly three decades to the Chinese capital of Beijing. A few months before that historic trip, appendicitis requiring immediate surgery struck *New York Times* reporter James Reston, who was in China preparing for

the president's visit. Instead of administering pharmaceutical anesthetics, his Chinese surgeons used acupuncture to control the pain during and following the
procedure. Reston wrote extensively about the successful and pain-free operation, fascinating readers in this
country and throughout the West.

Ever since, the acceptance of both Asian philosophies
and the methods they employ to maintain health—especially herbs and other natural substances—has been
growing among westerners. In 1992, the U.S. National
Institutes of Health, the federal government's largest
supporter of medical research, announced the establish-
ment of the Office of Alternative Medicine. Its goal remains to explore approaches to such chronic diseases as
allergies, arthritis, heart disease, and others for which
conventional Western medicine offers limited treatment
options. The decision to open the office stemmed in
part from the mounting evidence that increasing numbers of Americans seek alternative care every year for a
whole host of minor and major illnesses.

Among the most popular alternatives—and the ones
under a great deal of scrutiny by modern Western scientists—is the use of plants and plant material as medicine. Echinacea for colds, ginseng for anxiety and other
conditions, and now ginkgo biloba are just a few of the
remedies that fall under the rubric of "herbal medicine."

Understanding Herbal Medicine

The use of herbs has been integral to the practice of
medicine since the beginning of man's time on earth. In
fact, the word "drug" comes from the old Dutch word
drogge, meaning "to dry," as pharmacists, physicians,
and ancient healers often dried plants for use as medi-

cines. Today, approximately 25 percent of all prescription drugs are still derived from trees, shrubs, or herbs. Interestingly enough, the World Health Organization noted in 1985 that of 119 plant-derived pharmaceutical medicines, about 74 percent are used in modern medicine in ways that correlate directly with their traditional uses as plant medicines. (Ginkgo is a perfect example of this trend, since its first use as a "tonic for the brain" back in 2,800 B.C. remains its primary use today.)

The word "herb" as used in herbal medicine (also known as botanical medicine or, in Europe, as phytotherapy or phytomedicine) means a plant or plant part that is used to make medicine or aromatic oils for soaps and fragrances. An herb can be a leaf, a flower, a stem, a seed, a root, a fruit, bark, or any other plant part used for its medicinal property. (To date, only about 5,000 of the estimated 250,000 to 500,000 plant species have been extensively studied for their medicinal applications, which means we may well hear of brand-new plant-based remedies in the future.)

Generally speaking, herbal medicines work in much the same way as do conventional pharmaceutical drugs. Herbs contain a large number of naturally occurring substances that work to alter the body's chemistry in order to return it to its natural state of health. Unlike purified drugs, however, plants and other organic materials contain a wide variety of substances and, hence, less of any one particular active alkaloid. Herbs are thus less likely to be toxic to the body than are most pharmaceutical products.

Another benefit of natural herbs is that they tend to contain combinations of substances that work together to restore balance to the body with a minimum of side effects. You'll see the evidence of this with respect to ginkgo biloba in Chapter 2, but another good example is the plant meadowsweet. Meadowsweet contains compounds similar to those in aspirin that act as anti-inflammatories. These compounds, called salicylates, often irritate the stomach lining. Unlike commercially prepared aspirin, however, meadowsweet also contains substances that soothe the gastric lining and reduce stomach acidity: It provides pain relief while protecting the stomach from irritation.

Herbs as medicine come in many forms. Whole herbs are plants or plant parts that are dried and then either cut or powdered. They can be used as teas or for a variety of products. Herbs may also come in tablet or capsule form, which offer consumers the convenience of taking the herbs without having to taste them. In the case of ginkgo and other herbs, a process called extraction also takes place, through which the most active and essential ingredients are isolated, concentrated, and standardized.

In Chapter 8, you'll find out exactly how modern herbalists prepare the ginkgo extract currently used as medicine, and what it means to you as a consumer. For now, however, we will explore with you the remarkable substances found within the leaves of this age-old tree, and show you how they work to restore health to your brain and your body.

Find Out More About . . .

. . . Ginkgo

Q. I've heard that ginkgo is a miracle cure against aging and Alzheimer's disease. Could that be true?

A. When it comes to "miracle cures" of any type, keep in

mind the old adage "If it sounds too good to be true, it probably is." Studies to date show that ginkgo biloba appears to be a very safe and effective treatment for a host of common chronic conditions, as well as a healthy "tonic" for the brain that can stimulate memory and boost concentration. It will NOT, however, keep you young forever or cure you of all ills. Taking ginkgo may help your memory and concentration in the short term, and help certain body systems function more efficiently. However, to stop—or at least slow down—the aging clock and maintain optimal health, you've got to pitch in and do your part as well. That means eating a balanced and wholesome diet, exercising your body and mind on a regular basis, avoiding and alleviating stress as much as possible, sleeping well, and maintaining a vigilance about your health throughout your life.

In the chapters dealing with ginkgo's effects on specific illnesses and disorders (Chapters 3, 4, 5, 6, and 7), we give you information about the conditions ginkgo appears to benefit and show you the effects ginkgo has on the body systems involved. As you'll see, ginkgo's effects on the cardiovascular system and brain function are remarkable, and serve to alleviate many chronic and common conditions. Nevertheless, it's important to understand the way mainstream medicine treats these disorders, as well as to take some responsibility for their development and treatment yourself. To that end, we also provide lifestyle tips that might help you prevent these problems from developing in the first place, or alleviate their severity if you're already dealing with them. In Chapter 8, "Healthy Aging: Body and Mind," we outline some of the self-help strategies you can take on your own to maintain optimal health.

To sum up, no single herb or remedy can keep you strong, healthy, and feeling as young as possible. To do so, you must make a commitment to maintaining an overall healthy lifestyle that includes eating well, exercising regularly, controlling stress levels, and finding joy in the life you lead. Supplementing that lifestyle with ginkgo biloba and other healthful, natural remedies will bolster your efforts and help you feel even better as you age.

Q. Ginkgo sounds like a medicine. Do I need to get a prescription for it?

A. No, you don't need a prescription for ginkgo—you can buy it in your local health food store and some pharmacies. In 1994, Congress passed the Dietary Supplement Health and Education Act (DSHEA), which stated that herbs like ginkgo are considered "dietary supplements," not drugs, and can therefore be marketed as long as no medicinal claim is made on the label. We'll discuss this issue in more depth in Chapter 8.

Q. Can anyone take ginkgo, or are there some people who shouldn't take it at all?

A. Although ginkgo is considered safe, like most herbal medicines, it is a powerful drug that effects several changes in the body once ingested. We discuss these effects in depth in Chapter 2, and also discuss side effects and contradictions further in Chapter 9. Before you take ginkgo, you should read these sections with care, as well as discuss the matter with your physician, especially if you are currently taking any medication. A special warning goes to those with any medical problems that affect the blood's ability to clot, or who take anticoagulants like Coumadin or even the common aspirin. Taking ginkgo under these circumstances may put your health at risk. If you have any questions, talk to your doctor *before* taking ginkgo.

. . . Alternative Medicine

Q. I don't know anything about the Chinese medical tradition from which ginkgo derives. Do I need to understand Eastern philosophy in order to use ginkgo?

A. Not at all. As Chapter 2 will explain, there are valid reasons for ginkgo's effectiveness within the modern Western medical construct. Scientists have identified ingredients within the herb that act on the brain, the circulatory system, and the immune system in quite specific and scientifically identifiable ways.

On the other hand, traditional Chinese medicine (often abbreviated TCM) is a fascinating philosophy that you might find interesting and inspiring. At its heart, TCM from which ginkgo's healing properties were first derived holds that all of humanity, and each individual human, is part of a larger creation—the universe itself. Each of us is subject to the same laws that govern all of nature: We exist as equals with the stars, plants, animals, trees, oceans, and soils. It is no accident that natural images come into play as you read about this philosophy. TCM refers to the flow of bodily fluids and energy as channels and rivers, and the state of the body as a whole in terms of natural phenomena: cold, heat, dampness, dryness, and wind.

According to Chinese philosophy, human beings represent the juncture between heaven and earth and are thus a fusion of cosmic and earthly forces. Indeed, human beings *are* nature, and as such are subject to the same cyclic patterns, the same ebbs and flows, as the seasons and the tides. The states of the universe, the planet, the nation, and each individual human body are all connected by a unified system known as the *Tao*, or the Way. According to the *Tao*, when any part of this unified whole becomes unbalanced, natural disasters, such as floods or droughts or human disease, may occur: What injures the earth injures each of us, and vice versa. And efforts to heal the human body work to foster the health and well-being of the entire universe.

Q. How does traditional Chinese medicine view diseases and their treatment?

A. It's more appropriate to start with a discussion of how TCM views health. In Chinese medicine, your ability to maintain a balanced and harmonious internal environment determines the state of your health. Internal harmony is expressed through the principle of yin-yang, in which two opposing forces have united to create everything in the universe. Yin has connotations of cold, dark, and wet, while yang is warm, bright, and dry. Yin is quiet, static, and inactive, while yang is dynamic, active, and expansive. In human beings, parts of the body are ascribed more yin or more yang qualities, as are all physiological processes and diseases.

According to TCM, yin-yang imbalance is at the root of all disease. Yin-yang can become disturbed when the flow of energy through the body—the energy known as qi (pronounced "chee")—is interrupted or blocked in some way. In Chinese medicine, qi is the energy essential for life. All of your body's functions are manifestations of qi, and your health is determined by a sufficient, balanced, and unimpeded flow of qi. Qi ensures bodily function by keeping blood and body fluids circulating to warm the body, fight disease, and protect the body from negative forces in the external environment.

Qi circulates through the body along a continuous circuit of pathways known as meridians. These meridians flow along the surface of the body and through the internal organs. When you are healthy, you have an abundance of *qi* flowing smoothly through the meridians and organs, which allows your body to function in balance and harmony. If *qi* becomes blocked along one of your meridians, however, the organ or tissue meant to be nourished by this energy will not receive the *qi* it needs. TCM practitioners restore health by first locating where in the body *qi* is blocked, and then releasing it by using one or more traditional treatment methods: acupuncture, herbs, and exercises. In this way, proper energy flow to the body is restored.

Clearly, a thorough discussion of Chinese medicine goes far beyond the scope of this book. We do provide you with a list of other books in the Resources section, should you decide to further pursue your interest.

Q. Is there a way to combine alternative medicine with modern medicine?

A. Absolutely. Indeed, both Eastern and Western philosophies of health have their strong points, and in an interdependent world in which sharing among cultures continues every day, the best possible outcome is a health care system that combines the best of both traditions. Herbal medicine is a perfect example. In the past, modern Western physicians have largely shunned the use of herbs, putting them in the same basket as old wives' tales and witch doctors' "magical potions." Today, scientists are taking a hard—and very scientific—look at ways to use herbs to provide gentler but more effective treatments for many chronic, hard-to-treat diseases and conditions. Their studies prove, time after time, that herbs *are* medicine, and that alternatives such as massage and acupuncture do ease symptoms and restore balance to the body, and usually without debilitating side effects. Fortunately, mainstream physicians are listening to the results of these studies and starting to suggest herbal remedies—such as ginkgo biloba—to augment or even replace traditional prescriptions.

It should be noted that Asians, too, are making use of Western technological and pharmacological advances. Many Asian pharmacies stock both Eastern and Western medications, and many Asian patients now use a combined approach. Boundaries between the two traditions are dissolving, and both consumers and practitioners of health care are realizing the benefits of an integrated approach.

CHAPTER 2

The Tree of Health

Qi. In Chinese medicine, it is the source of energy necessary to sustain all life. It flows through meridians—energy passageways leading to every part of the body—bringing with it the "stuff" that enlivens the body. *Qi* also allows for and is represented by all physical and mental activities, including circulation, digestion, respiration, thinking, and feeling. When *qi* cannot reach all parts of the body, when something prevents *qi* from nourishing and activating the organs and tissues necessary to sustain health, disease is the result. Health is restored when one or more treatments—including consuming an herb like ginkgo—releases the blockage and allows *qi* to flow unimpeded.

From a Western medical perspective, of course, the idea of such a life-sustaining force does not exist. The human body is no more than the sum of its physiological parts, and what sustains life are very physical constituents like oxygen, hormones and other biochemicals, vitamins, and minerals that each cell, tissue, and organ needs in order to function.

On the other hand, there are some parallels we can

draw between Eastern and Western views of health and disease. For one thing, blood vessels and meridians look to be very similar, at least on the surface. Blood vessels carry oxygen and other nutrients, and nerve pathways carry certain hormones (called neurotransmitters), and these conduits bring life-sustaining "stuff" to all the cells and tissues of the body. Just like the meridians that carry *qi*, blood vessels and nerve tissue carry substances that both nourish the cells and trigger all processes of life, from digestion to respiration to the creation of thought and expression of feelings.

And, not unlike Chinese practitioners, our doctors look at disease as the result of an interruption of these normal healthful processes. In some cases, the interruption takes place because an external pathogen—a virus or bacteria—infects the body. In other cases, the body's own cells become corrupted and malfunction, as occurs with cancer.

Often, however, the pathways become blocked and the target cells and tissues never receive the nutrients and messages they need to function in a healthful way. Indeed, many of our most common chronic and acute conditions involve a disruption in either the circulatory system (the system of blood vessels, with the heart at its center) or the nervous system (the system of nerve fibers and chemicals, with the brain at its center). Heart disease and stroke, depression and Alzheimer's disease, certain common vision and hearing problems, even impotence and premenstrual syndrome can all be traced to a "blockage" of sorts in one or both of the body's pathways.

Modern medical science has made great strides in understanding the reasons why such blockages occur. Heredity almost always has a role to play, as does—to a lesser degree—the normal aging process. As you'll see, however, you are not powerless: What you eat, how much you exercise, and your ability to relax all have an impact on how well your body functions, and how clear those pathways remain.

In any case, it's important for you to understand another parallel between East and West: No single organ or system within the body works in isolation, nor are you as a single human being unaffected by the environment around you. You'll see, for instance, that your brain, which is part of the nervous system, requires nutrients and oxygen brought to it by the cardiovascular system. When something goes wrong with the heart and/or blood vessels, then, the brain may not function as it should. As for the environment affecting your health, there is no doubt that the toxins in the air you breathe and the food you eat have a negative effect on the way your body functions—or, on the other hand, that increasing the amount of beneficial minerals, vitamins, and fiber you consume can help improve your health. Nor, indeed, is there any doubt that the act of creating—from filling in a crossword to writing your memoirs—or learning something new every day from the world around you will significantly add to your vitality and strength. The idea that everything is connected, and that life and health exist within a cycle and have cycles of their own, are important concepts to keep in mind as you read this book.

THE CIRCULATION CONNECTION

As is true of so much in life, proper communication and timely delivery of essential goods and services is crucial to the health of the human body. Ginkgo biloba's primary attribute is its remarkable ability to ease communication between cells and deliver oxygen and other nutrients throughout the body. It does so by acting on two major systems of the body: the nervous system and the cardiovascular system. Before we discuss how this herb is able to exert such effects, it's important to gain an understanding of the systems involved.

The Nervous System

The human brain and nervous system form a vast communications network, more impressive even than the World Wide Web. Every emotion we feel, action we take, and physiological function performed is processed through the brain and nerve fibers that extend down the spinal cord and throughout the body.

The brain itself is divided into several large regions, each responsible for certain activities—a fact we'll explore at more length when we discuss Alzheimer's disease in Chapter 3. It is made up of billions of neurons (brain cells) that communicate with each other, and with nerve cells throughout the body, through a complex interaction.

Each neuron contains three important parts: the central body, the dendrites, and the axon. Messages from one cell enter the cell body of another through the dendrites, branchlike projections extending from the cell body. Once the central cell body processes the message, it can then pass on the information to its neighboring neuron through a cablelike fiber called the axon. At speeds faster than you can imagine, information about every aspect of human physiology, emotion, and thought zips through the body from one neuron to another in precisely this manner.

But there's a hitch: The axon of one neuron does not attach directly to its neighboring nerve cell. Instead, a tiny gap separates the terminal of one axon from the dendrites of the neuron with which it seeks to communicate. This gap is called the synapse. For a message to make it across a synapse, it requires the help of neurotransmitters, chemicals stored in packets at the end of each nerve cell. When a cell is ready to send a message, its axon releases a certain amount and type of neurotransmitter. This chemical then diffuses across the synapse to bind to special molecules, called receptors, which sit on the surfaces of the dendrites of the adjacent nerve cell. When a neurotransmitter couples to a receptor, it is like a key fitting into a starter that triggers a biochemical process in that neuron.

Scientists have named 40 to 50 neurotransmitters and believe at least 50 more are yet to be identified. Each must be present in sufficient amounts for the brain and nervous system to function properly. When too much or too little exists, or if the cells are unable to use the chemicals properly—when a "blockage" occurs somewhere along the lines of transmission—physical and/or psychological disease may develop. Depression, certain aspects of Alzheimer's disease and dementia, Parkinson's disease, and a host of other disorders involve a disruption of this system.

There remains a great deal we don't know about the brain and its functions, but scientists continue their research in laboratories around the world. One area of investigation is ginkgo biloba and its effects on the brain and nervous system. Early results indicate that it may play an important role in both reestablishing proper communication between neurons and improving the circulation of blood, oxygen, and nutrients throughout the brain. Again, the nervous system and the cardiovascular system are intricately linked.

The Cardiovascular System

Your cardiovascular system is made up of a vast network of blood vessels with a hollow muscular pump—the heart—at its center. The heart and blood vessels act as a single system, the purpose of which is to deliver oxygen and nutrients to body organs and to remove waste products from tissue cells. Blood, a fluid produced largely in bone marrow, carries these substances. The pumping action of the heart and the constant contraction and release of the blood vessels keep the blood in circulation.

Ten and a half pints of blood circulate through your body, bringing to each cell the oxygen, nutrients, and chemical substances necessary for its proper functioning and, at the same time, removing waste products. The blood consists of two basic parts: the formed cells (corpuscles), and the fluid plasma in which they are carried. Most blood cells are red cells, and their major function is to carry oxygen from the lungs to other parts of the body. Their red color comes from the pigment hemoglobin, which combines with oxygen and carries it in the blood.

For every 500 red cells in the circulating blood, there is a white cell, or leukocyte. Leukocytes, of which there are five types, are the body's main defense against disease and a wide variety of foreign invaders. They are intimately involved in the inflammatory response to injury and trauma, as well as in the allergic response to substances the body recognizes as enemies.

Finally, there are the platelets, tiny colorless disks. Together with the blood vessel walls and substances in the plasma called coagulation factors, platelets form the body's blood-clotting mechanism. They are the major protection of the body against continued bleeding when a blood vessel is damaged or severed.

Carrying all of these components through the body in a continuous circuit is the vascular system. It is divided into two components: the arteries, which deliver oxygen and nutrients from the heart to the body, and the veins, which bring deoxygenated blood back to the heart, where the cycle begins again. Both the arteries and the veins branch off into ever smaller and thinner-walled vessels, collectively called the "microcirculation." The arterioles conduct blood from the arteries to the capillaries, the smallest blood vessels that transmit oxygen and nutrients to the individual body cells. Deoxygenated blood and waste products flow first to venules (the smallest veins), which then pass blood along to veins back to the heart.

An interruption in the proper flow of blood through the meridians of the cardiovascular system usually occurs in one of two related ways: The vessels become too narrow and their walls too brittle or leaky, and/or the blood itself forms abnormal clots. These clots can then stick to the walls of the vessels (thereby narrowing them further) or become lodged in a vessel, blocking the passage of blood. Let's look briefly at each of these processes:

Arteriosclerosis: Most cases of cardiovascular disease involve arteriosclerosis, a condition in which the inner walls of the arteries harden and thicken, largely due to deposits of fatty substances. These substances form a plaque, which in turn causes a narrowing of the arteries. Over time, plaque can block the arteries and interrupt blood flow to the organs and tissues they supply, including the heart, brain, and extremities.

Abnormal blood clotting: Blood coagulation, or blood clotting, is a complex process that involves platelets, coagulation factors, and blood vessels. It represents our primary defense against excess bleeding and is an essential part of maintaining health. Diseases such as hemophilia (the lack of certain coagulation factors) and thrombocytopenia (the lack of sufficient platelets) are disorders of blood coagulation that occur when the blood fails to clot in a normal way.

At the same time, however, blood can form clots that contribute to arteriosclerosis and other forms of cardiovascular disease. High levels of circulating glucose (blood sugar) and insulin (a hormone produced in response to glucose)—hallmarks of the common chronic disease called diabetes—cause platelets to become more "sticky" and thus likely to form clots. Under certain circumstances, cholesterol, a fatlike substance, can attract blood cells to form plaques that stick to and narrow vessel walls, contributing to the process of arteriosclerosis.

In addition, platelets frequently form clots in response to damage to the inner arterial walls. As we'll discuss further in Chapter 5, this damage can come from many sources: High blood pressure pushes against arterial walls with greater-than-normal force and thus damages the lining. Toxic substances such as nicotine and asbestos irritate and damage the arterial lining. Certain hormones released during periods of high stress also have an abrasive effect.

Interestingly enough, ginkgo biloba contains substances that act on both the artery walls and the platelets to help keep the cardiovascular system clear and free to deliver the oxygen and nutrients necessary for health. Finding natural ways to do so has become urgent: Cardiovascular disease has become the nation's number-one killer.

The Culprits

Poorly communicating nerve cells, blocked arteries and veins, sticky blood cells . . . These conditions are responsible for some of the most common and debilitating medical conditions, including not only cardiovascular disease but Alzheimer's disease and other dementias, allergies, headache, impotence, and others.

Although each condition has its own set of specific causes, which we'll discuss in later chapters, there are some common threads that link them.

- *Heredity.* As scientists continue to discover every day, your genetic makeup—the characteristics you inherit from your parents—plays a definite, and sometimes crucial, role in your chances of developing certain diseases and disorders.
- *Lifestyle.* What you eat, how much (or if) you exercise, the quality of your sleep, and how you deal with stress all have a direct impact on the health of your nervous system and cardiovascular system.
- *Free-radical exposure.* One of the ways that blood vessels become damaged and tissue destroyed is through the action of free radicals. Free radicals are molecules that contain one or more unpaired electrons in their orbits. These unstable molecules, in an attempt to stabilize themselves, try to combine with nonradical cells in the body. By doing so, they often damage cell membranes as well as the internal structures of cells, including the genetic material encoded in DNA, the cell's genetic blueprint.

If we have too many free radicals in the body, disease can develop. Arteriosclerosis, which is involved in many diseases like heart attacks, stroke, peripheral vascular disease, and others, is affected by free radicals in many ways. Scientists also believe that free radicals cause or exacerbate degenerative brain disorders, like Alzheimer's disease and Parkinson's disease.

• *Inflammatory process.* Inflammation—your body's response to injury or invasion by internal or external enemies—can contribute to a host of medical problems if it occurs on a chronic basis. A substance released during the inflammatory process, called platelet-activating factor, or PAF, appears to be a main culprit. PAF is a body chemical that initiates or accelerates blood clotting, turning blood into a jellylike substance that does not flow easily. In addition to its direct effects on the cardiovascular system, the actions of PAF can also ultimately cause damage to nerve cells.

GINKGO BILOBA: THE EFFECTS

Starting in the 1930s, modern medicine began taking notice of the ginkgo biloba tree, long known in the East as a healthful botanical. Interest surged after a group of German and Japanese scientists isolated certain substances from ginkgo leaves they named "ginkgoglides" or "terpene lactones." Later, other researchers identified another group of chemicals they called "flavone glycosides." These two components are the substances in ginkgo that provide the wide range of benefits we now associate with this remarkable herb. Let's examine them one by one.

Flavone glycosides. These chemicals are part of the family of flavonoids. Flavonoids are the group of substances that give fruits and vegetables their bright colors, taste, and aromas. Better known as antioxidants, flavonoids—including ginkgo's glycosides—"clean up" excess free radicals, thereby protecting cells and tissues from damage. Flavonoids have varying antioxidant activity, and certain flavonoids seem to have an affinity for certain tissues. The flavonoids in ginkgo, for instance, reduce the "stickiness" of platelets in the blood as well as increase the strength of capillary walls. They also reduce inflammation, further protecting the body from disease.

Terpene lactones. These substances, of which scientists have isolated four types in ginkgo leaves, help to further offset processes that lead to the formation of unwanted blood clots. They tend to enhance the body's ability to use glucose and thus lower levels of circulating insulin. This protects against nerve cell damage as well as blood clotting. The terpene lactones also inhibit the actions of platelet-activating factor, thereby reducing the inflammatory response during allergy attacks.

In the late 1950s, Dr. Willmar Schwabe of the Schwabe Company in West Germany created an extract from the leaf that contains 24 percent flavone glycosides and 6 percent terpene lactones. As we'll discuss in greater depth in Chapter 9, this 24-to-6 ratio has become the standard formula for ginkgo biloba extract, which we will refer to as GBE from here on.

GBE has three main effects on the body: (1) It improves the quality and quantity of the circulation, which in turn improves circulation in the vital tissues and organs, such as the heart, brain, ears, and eyes; (2) it helps stop the damage to organs from free radicals; and (3) it blocks PAF. It does so because its unique ingredients perform several different functions within the body. These include:

- *Antioxidant.* Compounds in the plant can inactivate free radicals, the reactive toxic chemicals that can cause damage to cell membranes, proteins, and DNA. In addition, by protecting cell walls from damage from reactive compounds that would make them brittle, ginkgo helps make blood vessel walls more flexible and less likely to leak.
- *Anticoagulant.* Ginkgo has been shown to be an impressive blood thinner. It helps to keep red blood cells more pliable, allowing them to squeeze through small capillaries and venules. It also helps to inhibit the tendency for red blood cells and platelets to stick together and to adhere to blood vessel walls, which complicates arteriosclerosis.
- *Vasodilator.* GBE acts on the lining (endothelium) of the blood vessels and the system that regulates blood vessel tone. It does so by stimulating the release of certain chemicals that cause the contraction and relaxation of blood vessels. In essence, GBE stimulates greater tone in the venous system, thereby aiding in the dynamic clearing of toxic waste products that accumulate, especially with ischemia (insufficient oxygen supply).
- *Anti-inflammatory.* The ginkgolides have been shown to be potent inhibitors of platelet-activating factor, which means that GBE can alleviate bronchial spasm and other allergy symptoms. GBE has also been shown to prevent PAF from binding to platelets and thus prevent a whole range of undesirable cardiovascular effects such as arteriosclerosis, coronary artery disease, and stroke.
- *Neurotransmitter activator.* In addition to GBE's ability to increase the functional capacity of the brain via the mechanisms described above, namely as an antioxidant and anticoagulant, it also appears

to normalize certain chemical processes that take place between nerve cells. It appears to do so by normalizing or boosting the levels of certain neurotransmitters, including dopamine, serotonin, and acetylcholine—chemicals involved in such diseases as Alzheimer's disease, Parkinson's disease, and depression.

GINKGO BILOBA: THE STUDIES

As you can see, the leaves of the ginkgo biloba tree contain powerful chemicals that have remarkable healthful effects on the body. But there is still much we do not understand about the herb and the way it acts upon the systems of the body. To date, scientists have conducted at least 44 human studies and hundreds of animal studies involving ginkgo biloba extract. By and large, they've found that GBE does indeed have beneficial effects on a variety of body systems, and that when taken in average doses, rarely produces side effects.

That said, it's important to keep the information you read about ginkgo biloba—or any other "cure," for that matter—in perspective. Our understanding of disease, health, and treatment represents an ongoing process, and changes as new information becomes available. New attributes are being ascribed to aspirin, a medication that's been studied and been in widespread use for more than five decades. Research into the use of herbs like ginkgo biloba within a conventional Western medical context is in its infancy, and results of early tests may or may not be confirmed as time goes on.

You may remember the study we quoted at the beginning of Chapter 1 about ginkgo biloba's effects on

Alzheimer's disease patients. This study, conducted by a group of six physicians working under the auspices of the North American EGB Study Group, was designed to assess the safety and effectiveness of ginkgo in Alzheimer's disease and dementia caused by a certain kind of stroke. Their findings—that ginkgo improved the cognitive function of a majority of those studied—are now being explored further by other scientists. As is true for all preliminary research, there are still questions about methodology and results that require further investigation. This is especially true in the United States with its strict regulatory agencies.

As you can see, it isn't easy—even for professional and dedicated research scientists—to evaluate the meaning and validity of medical studies. Nevertheless, not a day goes by when you don't find a headline proclaiming a new cure or other development coming out of yet another research lab. That's why it's very important that you take the time to do further research—as you're doing by reading this book—about any new treatment that interests you, and to discuss the matter with your doctor.

Right now, we want to introduce you to some of the studies performed so far on ginkgo. Their results indicate that GBE exerts powerful effects on the body—literally from head to toe. Take a look:

The Brain (see Chapter 3)

Without question, GBE appears to have its greatest effect on the brain, stimulating concentration, reducing memory loss, and alleviating symptoms of Alzheimer's disease and other types of senile dementia. It does so by increasing blood flow to the brain, as well as boosting the action of neurotransmitters.

- A 1992 review of more than 40 clinical studies, published in the *British Journal of Clinical Pharmacology*, showed that GBE is effective in reducing loss of concentration, memory loss, and symptoms of senility. Although the positive results were greater in those people with existing impairments in this area, GBE also appears to help healthy young people as well.
- In a double-blind study published in a 1986 issue of the *International Journal of Clinical Pharmacology Research*, the reaction time in healthy young women performing a memory test improved significantly after the administration of GBE.
- A 1996 study published in the British journal *Life Science* shows that GBE inhibits the activity of monoamine oxidase, an enzyme involved in depression.

The Cardiovascular System (see Chapters 4 and 6)

Ginkgo improves blood flow to the heart, reduces stickiness of blood cells, and helps keep blood vessels strong and pliable. This can affect the heart, the brain (in the case of strokes), and the extremities, particularly the legs' resistance to a disease called peripheral vascular disease or intermittent claudication. GBE has also been shown to help treat impotence by increasing blood flow to the penis, as well as to alleviate symptoms of premenstrual syndrome by removing fluid from the breast and abdominal area more efficiently, thereby reducing tenderness and bloating. Here are a few of the studies that show how ginkgo affects the cardiovascular system:

- A study, published by the American Botanical Council in 1990, showed that GBE improved intermittent claudication—a disease caused by insufficient blood flow to the legs. Elderly patients who took GBE increased their pain-free walking distance from 30 to 100 percent.
- According to a 1965 study in the German journal *Arzneimittel-Forschung,* GBE lowered blood pressure and dilated peripheral blood vessels in 10 patients who had previously suffered a stroke, reducing swelling that otherwise may have caused permanent brain damage.
- A 1991 study in the *Journal of Sex Education and Therapy* studied two groups of men with impotence related to a lack of sufficient blood flow. The first group had previously responded to conventional therapies, while the other group had remained impotent. After six months of taking GBE, all of the men in the first group and nearly 75 percent of the men in the second group regained proper function.
- A 1993 study in *Gynecology and Obstetrics* (France) shows that GBE can be effective in alleviating breast tenderness and bloating related to premenstrual syndrome.

The Senses (see Chapter 7)

With arteriosclerosis and other age-related changes, blood flow to the ears and eyes may occur. Macular degeneration, a devastating eye disease that is the cause of most cases of adult-onset blindness, is one such disease. Dizziness, vertigo, and balance problems—at any age—may also be caused by decreased blood flow. We discuss this further in Chapter 7. Here are a few studies:

- Tinnitus: A 1986 French study published in *Presse Medicale* showed that ginkgo biloba extract improved the condition of all patients who had recent-onset tinnitus.
- Macular degeneration: A 1991 German study published in the journal *Klinische Montatsblatterfur Augenheilkunde* showed that by maintaining blood flow to the retina, GBE inhibits deteriorating vision in the elderly.
- A 1986 double-blind study in *Presse Medicale* found that 70 patients with vertigo of unknown origin benefited from taking GBE. At the end of the study, 47 percent of the patients treated with GBE were better, as opposed to just 18 percent of those who took a placebo.

As you can see from this impressive roster of well-conducted studies, taking GBE could be one of the best things you can do for your health. It may help to prevent certain chronic diseases from taking hold or progressing, as well as alleviate the symptoms of those you've already developed. You may also want to try it for the simple but elegant little "boost" it may give to your day-to-day ability to concentrate and focus. Chapter 3 will explore ginkgo's effects on the brain in more depth.

Find Out More About . . .

. . . The Circulation Connection

Q. My father just had a stroke and is having difficulty finding the right word when he's trying to speak. Is stroke a neurological disorder or a cardiovascular problem? And can ginkgo help him?

A. A stroke is a perfect example of how interrelated the systems of the body really are. A problem in the cardiovascular system—and we'll talk more about what kinds of cardiovascular problems can cause a stroke in Chapter 3—prevented a part of your father's brain from getting the oxygen and nutrients it needs to survive, and thus certain neurons are no longer able to communicate with one another, causing your father's speech problems.

As for whether ginkgo might be helpful to your father's condition, there is every reason to think that it might. GBE increases blood flow to the brain, thereby helping nourish parts of the brain that the injury to the vessels may have denied. It can also help protect against future problems by acting as a powerful antioxidant and blood vessel strengthener.

Q. What other kinds of patients benefit from taking ginkgo biloba for their circulation?

A. As we've discussed, circulation is crucial to the healthy functioning of every system and organ of the body—and so the examples of people who can gain from taking GBE are legion. Here are just a few:

• Nancy Hobbs, 56, suffers from Raynaud's disease, a disorder that causes her hands and feet to become abnormally cold and painful when exposed to the cold. Taking ginkgo for six weeks before going on vacation helped her to be able to enjoy skiing with her family instead of spending all her time in the lodge.

• Ray, 33, has had tinnitus—ringing in his ears—for several years. No other treatment helped until he started to take GBE. After a few months, he noticed a significant improvement in the symptoms, though the condition persists.

• Betty, 76, told her doctor that she felt that her memory had been slipping in recent months. After the doctor ruled out possible medical conditions, such as Alzheimer's disease and stroke, Betty started taking GBE. Not only has her memory improved somewhat, she also feels as if she has more day-to-day energy and vitality.

. . . Free Radicals

Q. I've heard a lot about free radicals and their relationship to disease. Where do they come from? And how do they damage the body?

A. When certain types of fats, oils, and other substances are exposed to oxygen, they become oxidized. This oxidized substance is called a free radical, and it seems to be at the root of a lot of cellular damage. Immune system function, metabolism, cell communication, and even the production of collagen, the substance that forms connective tissue like skin, all produce free radicals as a by-product of their processes.

In addition to free radicals produced in the body, we come into contact with many free radicals through our breathing and ingestion of food. In every quart of air we inhale (which takes about 30 minutes), we expose our cells to one billion free radicals. Processed foods are epecially rich in free radicals. A fast-food hamburger, sitting under a warming light for hours so that its fat content is exposed to oxygen, is a veritable free-radical factory.

The damage done by a free radical goes beyond the first cell it attacks. Not only is that cell injured—its ability to reproduce and metabolize permanently impaired—but it too becomes a free radical, ready to ravage another healthy cell. This chain reaction may continue, deforming one cell after another. If the resulting damage occurs in the immune system, you become more vulnerable to infection; when it happens to cardiovascular tissue, your risk for stroke and heart attack rises.

Q. And what about antioxidants? Where do they come from, and how do they prevent disease?

A. Like the enemies they fight, antioxidants also come from both outside and inside the body. Indeed, the human body is a remarkably self-contained organism. In addition to an immune system that fights against viruses and bacteria, we also utilize antioxidants—enzymes, vitamins, and minerals—that mop up free radicals before they can do any harm. Superoxide dismutase, an enzyme found in the liquid part of cells, is an example of an endogenous antioxidant—a substance the body makes itself. Vitamins C and E, beta-carotene (a precursor of vitamin A), and the mineral selenium are among the antioxidants we receive from the foods we eat or in supplements.

Q. Is there a link between free radicals and aging?

A. Some scientists think that the body becomes more vulnerable to free radicals with advancing age: Not only do we produce more free radicals, we are less able to defend ourselves against them. Free radicals then batter our cell membranes and DNA. They clog the walls of our arteries, destroy brain cells, stiffen and deplete our muscles, and throw our immune systems out of kilter. The damage done to these tissues may lead to the development of several age-related diseases, including arteriosclerosis, cancer, and Alzheimer's disease. That's why it's important to limit your exposure to free radicals, to consume foods rich in antioxidants, as well as to take supplements like ginkgo biloba that will help further protect you.

. . . Medical Research

Q. I've never understood what a double-blind study is. Can you explain?

A. A double-blind study is an attempt to reduce the natural tendency of the mind to influence the results of a treatment. The study usually involves two sets of researchers and two sets of patients. The first set of researchers gives one group of patients a treatment—ginkgo biloba, in this case—and another group of patients a placebo (an inactive substance). No one involved knows which patients receive the ginkgo and which the placebo, including the researchers. Just to be on the safe side, however, another group of researchers evaluate the results. Especially when it comes to subjective observations, such as the improvement of memory or an increase in energy or boost in mood, it is especially important for both researchers and patients to be free of any potential bias. And, generally speaking, the results of double-blind studies are considered to be more accurate than those from other types of research protocol.

Q. I understand that many more tests studying the effects of ginkgo biloba have been done on rats and other animals than on humans. Can we assume that the results have some bearing on how ginkgo might affect humans?

A. Absolutely. Decades of research point to the strong likelihood that chemicals or other substances that cause or alleviate disease in well-designed animal studies will also do the same in humans. For instance, all 25 chemicals known to cause cancer in humans have also been shown to cause cancer in animals—and generally involving the same organs. Federal regulatory agencies often base their regulation on the predictive value of animal tests to human disease and treatment. On the other hand, before any drug can be marketed for use in humans, it must undergo thorough double-blind human testing. When it comes to ginkgo, you'll no doubt be hearing more about further human studies as research into the effects of this herb continues.

CHAPTER 3

Ginkgo and Your Brain

In Chapter 2, we mapped out the basic structure and function of the brain and nervous system. We hope you came away from that discussion with two things: an appreciation of the complexity and wonder of this amazing organ, and an understanding of the intimate relationship between the nervous system and the cardiovascular system. The brain could not function if the vast and intricate system of blood vessels were not bringing essential oxygen and nutrients to the brain's billions of neurons. It could not produce the chemicals it needs (the neurotransmitters) to send its messages within the structure of the brain and throughout the body. When insufficient blood flow to the brain occurs, or when neurotransmitters fail to properly send or receive the brain's messages, our ability to function becomes seriously impaired. Indeed, perception, memory, mood, movement, and behavior all depend on the power of the brain to fuel their activities.

During the 1990s—dubbed the Decade of the Brain by government agencies and scientists—advanced technology has allowed us to glimpse the complicated inner workings of the brain. We're beginning to understand how information coming into the brain is sorted and stored as memory, then retrieved at a later point. We know a little bit more about what "learning" something really means. For instance, it appears that information coming into the brain is broken down into separate processing streams and stored in various parts of the brain. They fit into roughly 20 categories that the brain uses to organize knowledge, including fruits and vegetables, animals, body parts, colors, numbers, letters, nouns, verbs, proper names, faces, facial expressions, several different emotions, and several different features of sound.

When we try to retrieve information about a particular object or word, we delve into one of these categories. But the items in these categories are not images of the items themselves, but rather a set of indexes that draw such information from other parts of the brain. Each specific realization or memory is achieved by processing in a different area of the brain. If you imagine your cat, for instance, you retrieve the image of the feel of her fur from one place in your brain, her name from another, and her color from another—and it all happens pretty much in the blink of an eye.

But no one has yet found any "place" where all the information comes together, presenting a whole picture of what is being felt, seen, or experienced. Clearly, however, awareness and subjectivity—how you feel about what you see and hear—and how well you remember what you've experienced and learned involve networks of millions of nerve cells throughout the brain. You can see how important it is that every part of the brain receive the nutrients it needs, and that messages pass between neurons quickly and efficiently.

Even when we're young and presumably at the top of

our game, there are times when the synapses in the
brain just don't spark as quickly as we'd like them to,
when the indexing processing goes a bit more slowly.
We can't quite find the "file" we need to recall a bit of
stored information or cannot concentrate on the new
tasks before us. Unfortunately, as the brain ages and
changes, these problems often become worse.

The Brain and Aging

Grandma Moses started painting at the age of 100,
completing 25 visions of New England after that birthday, and writer I. F. Stone mastered Greek in his 80s in
order to write a critique of Socrates. Clearly, these two
examples—and we bet you know of a few vital, creative
older people yourself—show that aging does NOT
mean automatically losing your ability to remember or
to learn. In fact, by repeatedly testing people over a
period of years, researchers from Penn State found in
1996 that intelligence did not necessarily decline with
age, but could actually increase as people got older. Dr.
Marilyn Albert, a neuropsychologist at Massachusetts
General Hospital in Boston, has found that while the
speed with which the brain processes information does
fall off with age, older people will do just as well as
younger people on a test of cognitive ability if given
enough time.

Nevertheless, it is true that certain age-related
changes do occur, and they may affect memory and
cognitive ability. From age 20 to age 70, the average
brain loses about 10 percent of its mass and shows mild
atrophy in certain portions of the brain that causes a
slowdown in reaction times. Tests measuring blood
flow to areas of the brain while people perform memory
tasks indicate that younger people exhibit more activity

in different areas of the brain—primarily the hippocampus and adjacent structures—when encoding new information than do elderly people. This lack of blood flow may help explain "ordinary" memory problems associated with aging as well as some aspects of degenerative brain disorders like Alzheimer's disease and Parkinson's disease.

Why blood flow fails to reach these structures in older people remains unknown, but narrowing and scarring of the blood vessels (arteriosclerosis) is a likely explanation in most cases. In specific disease processes, healthy tissue may become damaged by chronic exposure to toxic chemicals, or attacked by as yet unidentified viruses. Another possibility is that changes in the chemical makeup of neurotransmitters, or in the ability of neurons to recognize or transmit the messages they send, contribute to the problems.

How to keep the brain healthy and vital throughout the life span remains an area of intense study among researchers around the world. One subject under investigation is ginkgo biloba and its effects on blood vessels and neurotransmitters. Let's see how ginkgo works to improve brain function in several common conditions involving memory, learning, and mood.

CEREBRAL INSUFFICIENCY

Jenny is a 36-year-old office manager for a computer software company. In recent months, as the company has been working to put out a new product, Jenny has been spending 10 to 12 hours a day behind her desk. She gets very little exercise and has been concentrating mainly on very routine and tedious tasks, such as entering product codes into a database and cross-referencing mailing lists. Jenny recently visited her doctor complaining of an inability to concentrate, feelings of lethargy and distraction, and even physical weakness and dizziness. After ruling out potentially serious medical conditions, such as high blood pressure and heart disease, her doctor gave her a simple prescription: Get more exercise to improve circulation to the brain and take ginkgo biloba, an herb known for its properties as a cardiovascular and cerebral tonic.

Although we here in the United States rarely use the term, Europeans would diagnose Jenny as suffering from "cerebral insufficiency," which European medical doctors describe as a syndrome of 12 related symptoms: difficulties in concentration and memory, distraction, confusion, lethargy, fatigue, weakness, depression, anxiety, dizziness, ringing in the ears, and headache. In this book, we'll be looking separately at many of these problems—depression and other mood disorders, dizziness, and ringing in the ears—as well as those conditions most related to the aging brain, specifically Alzheimer's disease and other dementias.

But it appears that even healthy young people like Jenny can lack "brainpower" at certain points in their lives—and for a variety of reasons, usually related to lifestyle. Lack of regular, vigorous exercise to maximize blood flow is perhaps the most obvious one. Sleep deprivation is another, for sleep restores not only the body but the brain as well. Eating a fat-rich, nutrient-poor diet can start the process of arteriosclerosis in childhood, so that by age 35 or 40, the effects on blood flow in the brain can already be significant.

Fortunately, it's never too early—or late—to incorporate healthy habits into your life. In Chapter 8, we outline some diet, exercise, and stress-relieving strategies for you to consider. In the meantime, one helpful addition to your daily regimen appears to be ginkgo biloba. Not only will it help boost your brainpower, but it acts as an antioxidant to protect your blood vessel and tissue health throughout your life span.

Ginkgo and Brain Vitality

As mentioned in Chapter 2, GBE can improve your mental performance no matter what your age. In a double-blind study conducted at the Laboratory of Physiology in Paris, the results of which were published in a 1986 *Presse Medicale*, for instance, eight healthy young women aged 25 to 40 were given either a placebo or 120, 240, or 600 milligrams of GBE. One hour later, they were subjected to a battery of highly sophisticated and reliable tests of short-term memory. Those who had taken 600 mg GBE scored far higher than those who had taken the placebo did—and experienced no side effects. So in addition to protecting your brain from long-term damage and helping to keep tissues nourished and healthy, ginkgo also helps to improve short-term memory.

As you may remember from Chapter 2, GBE affects the brain in three main ways:

- *Increases blood flow to the brain.* GBE improves the ability of the blood vessels to deliver glucose—blood sugar that cells use as energy—because it keeps the vessels functioning properly, a matter we'll discuss at length in Chapter 4.
- *Strengthens brain cells.* By acting as a free-radical scavenger, GBE protects the tissues of the brain from harm. It strengthens cell membranes, thus preventing cellular damage.
- *Increases neurotransmission.* Studies show that

GBE activates the enzyme that exchanges sodium for potassium in red blood cells. This exchange improves the energy for electrical charge of the cell membrane, making transmission of nerve messages more effective.

Although these effects take on more importance in older people and in those with brain disease, GBE helps brain tissue at any age. Of course, taking GBE is just one way to get your blood pumping and your brain cells clicking away at top speed. For a list of other methods of protecting yourself today and for the future, see the prevention tips on pages 58–60.

ALZHEIMER'S DISEASE AND OTHER DEMENTIAS

Although losing mental capacity is perhaps the greatest fear associated with aging, the vast majority of people grow old without suffering any serious decline in their ability to remember or learn new facts. That said, in addition to the more minor problems associated with aging, about 15 percent of older people eventually do develop dementia, an organic brain disorder that interferes with their mental functions and that tends to grow worse with time. The incidence increases with age; about 50 percent of people over age 85 suffer some symptoms of dementia.

Of this number, approximately 50 to 60 percent—about 4 million men and women over age 65—suffer from a type of dementia called Alzheimer's disease (AD), while another 20 percent have vascular dementia, a condition in which a series of small strokes ("brain attacks") damages or destroys brain tissue. In essence, vascular dementia is the result of clots or bleeding within the brain. As a result, part of the brain is deprived of blood, which causes neurons to die. Whereas major strokes may cause a loss of movement in an arm or leg or interfere with speech and comprehension, these ministrokes cause subtle changes in the brain's higher intellectual capacities, including memory. (We'll discuss ginkgo's impact on cerebrovascular and cardiovascular health in more depth in Chapter 4.)

Alzheimer's disease, the most common dementia of aging, is a progressive disorder that primarily affects the cerebral cortex, the cap of deeply grooved tissue in which the brain's higher powers of cognition and memory are believed to be stored. It occurs when brain tissue is destroyed, forming neurofibrillary tangles and plaques made up of a toxic protein called beta amyloid. Research on the cause of AD continues, but no one knows for sure what triggers the destruction of brain tissue. Among several possible causes are genetic factors (AD tends to run in families), toxic exposures, abnormal protein production, viruses, and abnormalities in the barrier between the blood and the brain.

In 1997, a group of researchers at the University of South Florida directly linked the process of inflammation and blood vessel damage to Alzheimer's disease in a well-designed animal study. Published in the July 1997 issue of the *Journal of Submicroscopic Cytology and Pathology,* the study furthered a theory that AD may be an inflammatory disorder, possibly a result of the brain's fight against infection triggered by the beta amyloid plaques.

No matter what acts as the initial trigger, as the disease progresses, memory, speech, and other aspects of cortical functioning begin to diminish. Usually AD begins slowly, and the first symptoms are often simple forgetfulness: People with early-stage AD may have trouble recalling recent events, activities, or names of familiar people or things, and simple problems may become harder to solve. As the disease progresses, however, symptoms become more pronounced, prompting medical intervention. Routine tasks like dressing, bathing, and doing the dishes are forgotten. Talking, reading, and understanding become impossible. People with AD often suffer from anxiety, depression, and aggression.

Diagnosing Alzheimer's Disease

To date, no laboratory test exists that can diagnose Alzheimer's disease with any certainty. The only direct evidence is the presence of beta amyloid plaques, which can be viewed only at autopsy after the patient's death. At specialized centers, however, experienced doctors are able to diagnose AD correctly probably 80 to 90 percent of the time. They do so by first ruling out any other possible causes of the patient's memory and cognitive problems through a thorough medical exam, which may include laboratory blood and urine tests as well as a brain scan.

In addition, a series of neurological tests and quizzes can help identify a person suffering from AD. In 1997, a study published in the *Archives of Neurology* reported a new test that can identify patients with early stages of Alzheimer's disease in 90 percent of cases. The four quizzes probe a patient's ability to recall words and images seen moments before, along with the ability to solve a simple clock problem.

The first test simply asks a person to state the current year, month, date, day of the week, and approximate time. The next quiz involves flash cards, shown in sets of four, that picture ordinary objects in 16 different categories. After viewing the cards, the patient is asked to recall the picture sets. Reminder words are provided if needed. Few people can recall all of the categories, but a normal person will benefit from the reminder words. However, someone with Alzheimer's will not benefit from reminders. In the clock problem, a patient is given pencil and paper and asked to draw a clock face, with the 12 numbers in the proper place, and to arrange the hands to show a specific time—say, 20 minutes to four. People with memory problems will leave out numbers, arrange the hands in the wrong position, or put the numbers in the wrong position on the clock face. In the final quiz, a patient has one minute to name as many objects as possible in a single category, such as "vegetables" or "furniture." People with normal memories will easily come up with 12 or more.

Obviously, this is not a quiz you can, or should, take or evaluate at home, but it does reveal the profound changes in memory and cognition that come with Alzheimer's disease. Indeed, even the simplest tasks we take for granted every day become lost to the person with this devastating disease. Fortunately, slowly but surely, scientists are finding new ways to treat AD, and are increasingly looking toward a natural brain and cardiovascular booster called ginkgo biloba.

TREATING ALZHEIMER'S AND DEMENTIA

At this time, no treatment exists that will cure Alzheimer's disease or repair the damage done to the brain by cerebrovascular disease. Some medications (described later) may help improve symptoms and, perhaps, slow the progress of AD. Among the more promising treatments under investigation is ginkgo biloba, which appears to help improve symptoms of both types of dementia.

Ginkgo and Dementia

As discussed in previous chapters, several recent studies prove that daily doses of 120 to 240 mg of GBE lead to dramatic improvement in such symptoms of Alzheimer's disease as memory loss, loss of cognitive function, loss of attention span, disorientation, emotional instability, depression, anxiety, and loss of motivation—especially in people in the early stages of the disease.

GBE works its magic on the brain primarily by limiting free-radical damage on brain tissue and by increasing microcirculation in the tiny veins and arterioles throughout the brain, thereby allowing better delivery of oxygen and glucose to brain tissue. It also helps to stimulate the release and transmission of acetylcholine, a brain chemical in short supply in people with Alzheimer's disease.

Ginkgo's ability to inhibit the action of platelet-activating factor (PAF) may also play a crucial role. As you may remember from Chapter 2, PAF triggers the inflammatory process. Chronic inflammation makes blood vessels more brittle and leaky, leading to an increased risk of vascular dementia caused by many "ministrokes," and plays a direct role in damaging brain tissue in Alzheimer's disease. As you'll see, new studies linking aspirin and other conventional anti-inflammatories to AD prevention confirm ginkgo's positive effects in this regard.

Mainstream Medical Options

Only a few treatments prove successful in alleviating symptoms of AD. Low doses of antipsychotic medications, for instance, can sometimes help calm symptoms of anxiety and agitation as well as moderate the occurrence of hallucinations. In the early 1990s, scientists developed a new drug specifically for AD called tacrine (Cognex). This medication works by inhibiting the enzyme cholinesterase, which allows levels of acetylcholine to rise—very much the same way that GBE acts. About 30 percent of AD patients find that tacrine helps slow the progression of their memory loss. More recently, the medication donepezil (Aricept) has become available. It works just like tacrine but tends to cause fewer side effects. Developed in 1997, Aricept blocks the chemical breakdown of acetylcholine and thereby increases levels of the chemical within the brain. Although patients reported some gastrointestinal side effects such as diarrhea, nausea, and vomiting, a high percentage were able to tolerate the drug well.

Prevention Is the Best Medicine

Although no cure yet exists for Alzheimer's disease or dementia due to cerebrovascular damage, there are some preventative measures you can take. According to the Institute for Brain Aging and Dementia, the following factors may contribute to the prevention of Alzheimer's disease and other dementias:

- *Pursue higher learning.* Once again, it's important to keep learning, and the younger you start challenging yourself, the better. People with at least eight years of education have a reduced risk of

Alzheimer's disease. Conversely, uneducated people have about twice the risk of developing dementia by age 75 as compared to those with an eighth-grade education or beyond. The reason? Synapses are strengthened by frequent use (called use-dependent plasticity). Research has shown that people who use language skills have larger and more intricate brain connections in the areas of the brain responsible for language. Even in those who are already victims of Alzheimer's disease, particular skills, such as reading, calculating, singing, playing the piano, drawing, and golf, remain intact when dementia is moderately advanced.

- *Keep moving.* According to the MacArthur Foundation, people over 75 years of age who exercise for approximately 30 minutes each day perform better on several cognitive function tests.
- *Use estrogen-replacement therapy.* Owing to the loss of estrogen at menopause, women in late life are at increased risk for stroke, heart disease, osteoporosis, and Alzheimer's disease. The Women's Health Initiative and the Alzheimer's Disease Cooperative Study Unit are currently investigating estrogen-replacement therapy's effect on the occurrence of dementia.
- *Boost your antioxidant intake.* Free radicals can damage brain cells and may contribute to the brain damage caused by Alzheimer's disease. Antioxidants help keep blood vessels and cell membranes strong, and thus can limit brain cell damage that may occur with vascular stroke and the AD degenerative process. Among those most useful for elderly patients, especially, are vitamins C and E, zinc, and selenium.
- *Take aspirin or other anti-inflammatories.* Studies

have shown that people taking an anti-inflammatory medicine, such as aspirin or ibuprofen, have a reduced risk of developing Alzheimer's disease. Those taking an anti-inflammatory agent and a type 2 histamine receptor blocker (found in anti-ulcer medication) have shown an even greater reduction in the risk of developing Alzheimer's disease.

- *Use it or lose it.* By stimulating the brain, education may establish more neuronal pathways early in life as well as prompt people to remain cognitively active throughout life. Even among people who led very active lives—by traveling, taking courses, reading—maintained intellectual function much longer than those who became couch potatoes did. Jigsaw puzzles and games like chess help to foster spatial orientation and stimulate inductive reasoning.

- *Maintain a healthy sense of self-esteem.* A study performed at the University of Southern California in Los Angeles found that people with stronger self-confidence showed much less of an increase in stress hormones when put in a stressful situation than did those who did not feel as confident.

In general, the message is fairly straightforward: Staying healthy and active, both physically and mentally, may well go a long way toward preserving your ability to think, dream, remember, and create as you grow older. A healthy diet rich in antioxidants and GBE supplements to improve circulation in the brain and the entire nervous system will only increase your chances that your golden years will be among the best of your life.

DEPRESSION

At any age, depression is one of the most common health problems in the United States today. According to the National Institute of Mental Health, more than one in 20 Americans—some 17.8 million people—suffer from depression every year. The personal costs of this disease are incalculable. It is a disease that robs the spirit of life and the body of energy. Measured by days spent in bed and body pain experienced, depression ranks second only to advanced heart disease in exacting a physical toll. A 1989 study published by the *Journal of the American Medical Association* reported that depression is more isolating than any other chronic illness.

Depression does not discriminate. The disorder affects people of every age, race, religion, and culture. It is neither an inevitable side effect of aging nor a disorder reserved for the young and stereotypically self-indulgent. In fact, each of us is more or less vulnerable to the disease, depending on a variety of factors. There appears to be a genetic component to depression, since people with a family history of the disease are at higher risk. Women tend to be more prone to depression than men, although new research indicates that men with depression may exhibit different symptoms, such as aggression and substance abuse, and thus are misdiagnosed. Incidence of depression also increases with age, owing probably in equal part to age-related physical changes in the body and brain and one's response to those changes. In addition, dealing with the loss of loved ones, coping with chronic illness, and losing one's independence also have an impact on mental and emotional health.

In any case, it is important to recognize that depression is not merely a "blue mood," but a medical disorder that can affect your physical as well as your mental health. To give you an idea of how wide-ranging its effects can be, here is a list of common symptoms of depression:

Signs and Symptoms of Depression

- A persistent sad, anxious, or "empty" mood
- Sleeping too little or too much, or early awakening
- Reduced appetite and weight loss, or increased appetite and weight gain
- Loss of interest and pleasure in activities once enjoyed
- Persistent physical symptoms—especially gastrointestinal problems, headaches, and pain—that don't respond to treatment
- Difficulty concentrating, remembering, or making decisions
- Fatigue or loss of energy
- Feelings of guilt and worthlessness
- Thoughts of death or suicide

Depression can be triggered both by emotional trauma and underlying psychological problems. It can also lead to, or result from, difficulties in coping with family, career, and personal challenges. However, in this book, we focus on the biological causes and treatment of depression, since that's how ginkgo biloba fits into the picture.

Where Is Mood?

Located on top of the brain stem and buried under the cerebral cortex is a set of structures called the limbic system. Scientists believe that this highly complex—and still largely unmapped—region is "home base" to our emotions. It receives and regulates emotional information and helps govern sexual desire, appetite, and stress. Three main centers of the limbic system are the thalamus-hypothalamus, the hippocampus, and the amygdala. The thalamus-hypothalamus forms a kind of "brain within a brain," regulating a variety of processes, including appetite, thirst, sleep, and certain aspects of mood and behavior. The hippocampus and the amygdala help create memory as well as gauge emotions.

Scientists have also been able to trace how the limbic system registers emotion and then produces emotional reactions in cooperation with other parts of the brain and body. Studies performed at the National Institute of Mental Health and published in the March 1995 issue of the *American Journal of Psychiatry* hint at the complexity of the process. These experiments show, for instance, that emotional opposites like happiness and sadness involve independent patterns of activity: When we feel happy, activity in the region of the cerebral cortex responsible for forethought and planning decreases dramatically, as does activity in the amygdala. When we're unhappy, on the other hand, the amygdala and another part of the cortex become more active.

When it comes to depression, the studies show that the same area of the brain—the left prefrontal cortex—appears to be involved in both depression and ordinary sadness, but in different ways. It becomes more active during ordinary sadness but almost completely shuts

down with depression. That might explain the empti-
ness and numbness many depressed people report.

What disturbs normal functioning of the brain—
what makes one part of the brain more active or inactive than usual—can usually be traced to an imbalance
of neurotransmitters, the nervous system's chemical
messengers. An imbalance of three neurotransmitters—
serotonin, norepinephrine, and dopamine—appears to
be involved in most cases of depression. These same
imbalances also occur in people who suffer from anxiety, eating disorders, obsessive-compulsive disorder,
and several other psychological disturbances.

Serotonin is the neurotransmitter scientists focus on
the most when it comes to depression. With the most
extensive network of any neurotransmitter, serotonin
influences a wide range of brain activities, including
mood, behavior, movement, pain, sexual activity, appetite, hormone secretion, and heart rate. People with depression have been found to have lower amounts than
usual of serotonin in the brain. Dopamine is another
neurotransmitter important in the disease of depression.
It follows two main pathways in the brain. One pathway connects to a portion of the brain called the corpus
striatum, which controls movement. When this pathway malfunctions, as it does in such disorders as Parkinson's disease and Huntington's chorea, problems
with muscle control arise. The other pathway connects
to the limbic system. When dopamine does not exist in
proper amounts or is unable to reach organs of the limbic system, emotional problems such as depression may
occur. Norepinephrine is the third neurotransmitter
thought to be involved in depression. Lower-than-nor-
mal amounts of norepinephrine have been measured in
people who are depressed. Since norepinephrine is part
of the body's stress response, this lowered level may

explain the decreased energy and ability to cope that accompanies depression.

TREATING DEPRESSION

In addition to psychotherapy to treat the underlying and resulting emotional challenges connected to depression, doctors now look toward drug therapy to treat this often stubborn disorder. In fact, prescriptions for antidepressants and stimulants by doctors increased dramatically from 1985 to 1994, according to a study published in the *Journal of the American Medical Association* on February 18, 1998. The number of visits during which a psychotropic medication was prescribed increased from 32.7 million to 45.6 million. We'll discuss the types of drugs that act to restore proper brain chemistry later. For now, let's see how ginkgo biloba works to help alleviate depression.

Ginkgo and Depression

Although ginkgo biloba is still under investigation as a treatment for depression, its effects on brain chemistry and brain circulation appear to benefit those who suffer from this disorder. In a double-blind study published in the German journal *Geriatric Forschung,* depressed patients who weren't responding well to antidepressant medications were given either GBE in dosages of 80 mg three times per day, or a placebo for eight weeks—and all stayed on their antidepressant medication as well. After four weeks, those taking GBE showed a 50 percent reduction in depression, and after eight weeks, the same group showed a 68 percent decrease in depression.

Ginkgo may act on the brain in two different ways to alleviate depression. First, it appears to boost the activity of certain neurotransmitters, including norepinephrine and acetylcholine. In addition, it also helps to increase circulation in the brain, which may be lower in depressed patients than in normal patients. In fact, depression is sometimes the earliest sign of dementia, and may signal the first symptoms of a brain gone awry due to decreased circulation. And although depression is probably caused by a combination of biological and environmental factors, ginkgo's effects on the brain certainly allow the body to do everything it can to fight debilitating depression.

GBE offers an added bonus for those already taking an antidepressant medication. A recent study demonstrated that GBE dramatically relieved antidepressant-induced sexual dysfunction in men and women taking a wide variety of antidepressant drugs. After just four to six weeks of twice-daily doses of GBE ranging from 60 to 120 mg, GBE alleviated erectile failure, anorgasmia (failure to reach orgasm), and diminished sex drive in 91 percent of the women and 76 percent of the men in the study, all of whom reported symptoms of sexual dysfunction after beginning antidepressant medication.

Mainstream Medications

Several types of drugs—each of which works to fine-tune the balance of neurotransmitters in a slightly different way—have been found to be most effective in treating depression: selective serotonin reuptake inhibitors (SSRIs), which, as their name implies, boost both the levels of serotonin and the ability of brain cells to use it; triçyclic antidepressants, which raise levels of both serotonin and norepinephrine; and monoamine oxidase inhibitors, which work to inhibit an enzyme (monamine oxidase) that breaks down norepinephrine and other neurotransmitters. Other drugs, such as buproprian (Wellbutrin), work by other mechanisms, as yet to be defined. In fact, scientists believe that ginkgo biloba may have some of the same effects of slowing down monoamine oxidase activity, and therefore boosting norepinephrine levels. However, there is no evidence that dietary restrictions are necessary with ginkgo, as they are with MAO-inhibitors.

Find Out More About . . .

. . . Ginkgo and Treatment of Other Brain Disorders

Q. I frequently suffer from headaches. Could taking GBE help me feel better?

A. Headaches may very well be the most common health complaint in all of history. For some they are an occasional annoyance, but for others headaches are either a part of daily life, or are periodic, completely debilitating conditions.

Finding the cause of a headache is no easy task, as any physician will tell you. A headache can be caused by many stimuli, including allergies, arthritis, depression, environmental pollution, diet, stress, exertion, glaucoma, hormone fluctuations, trauma, sinusitis, stroke, tumors, and visual problems. For some people, a couple of aspirin will do the trick. But for sufferers of chronic headaches, migraines, cluster headaches, or other treatment-resistant types of head pain, headaches can become a painful way of life.

And there are probably as many headache remedies out

there as there are headache causes. Aspirin, acetamino-
phen, and ibuprofen are some of the more common over-
the-counter remedies. Countless prescription remedies exist, from lidocaine nose sprays to Prozac. Herbal remedies
include feverfew, goldenseal, lavender, peppermint, rosemary, and, of course, GBE.

Ginkgo biloba is most likely effective on headache pain
because it is so effective at increasing circulation to the
brain. No matter what is causing a headache, the perfusion
of oxygen and glucose into the brain precipitated by
ginkgo biloba helps the brain to get back to its normal,
pain-free state. Once again, ginkgo biloba helps the body
to help itself.

Q. My mother was recently diagnosed with Parkinson's disease. Could taking GBE be helpful for her as well?

A. Since GBE apparently boosts the ability of brain cells to
communicate with one another and with nerve cells
throughout the body, there's a good chance GBE can help
your mother. Parkinson's disease involves the loss of the
crucial neurotransmitter dopamine, which helps trigger and
control muscle movement and other body functions. However, she should work closely with her doctor to manage
the disease with other medications, including preparations
of levodopa, which replaces the lost dopamine.

. . . Memory and Learning

Q. Besides increasing blood circulation through the brain, how
else might exercise improve memory and cognitive function?

A. An animal study performed at the University of California at Irvine revealed that treadmill exercise raises the levels of brain-derived neurotropic factor, or BDNF, a nerve growth factor that keeps neuron levels healthy. And the increase in BDNF occurred not just in motor areas of the brain but also in areas involved in memory, learning, and cognition.

Q. I've always heard that humans use only 10 percent of their brain. Is this true?

A. Although no one knows exactly what proportion of the brain we use, it is likely that it is significantly more than 10 percent. Think of it this way: If 90 percent of your brain were removed, you'd be left with a brain the size of a sheep's—not exactly the smartest animal on the farm. Furthermore, we know that damage to even a small area of the brain, like that caused by stroke, can cause devastating disabilities. Parkinson's disease, a degenerative brain disease, starts with damage to a portion of the brain the size of a quarter.

. . . Depression

Q. Can I stay on my antidepressant medication and take ginkgo, too?

A. In studies of depressed patients who showed improvement on GBE, antidepressant medication was continued throughout the study—and without any adverse side effects. In fact, as discussed earlier, the benefit of taking GBE with antidepressants is that the herb helps prevent the common side effect of sexual dysfunction in both men and women. As long as you talk to your doctor about taking the herb—you should tell him or her about every medication or supplement you consume—you shouldn't hesitate to add ginkgo biloba to your regimen. See Chapter 9 for more information.

Q. I've been taking St. John's wort to treat my depression. I feel better, but wonder if I can also take ginkgo at the same time. I like the fact that ginkgo also works to help stimulate memory.

A. You should feel free to take ginkgo along with St. John's wort, another age-old herb now in use to help elevate mood. Like ginkgo, it works by helping to inhibit monoamine oxidase and acting as a serotonin reuptake inhibitor. St. John's wort is also known to have antiviral and antibacterial effects. A plant native to many parts of the world, including the United States, where it grows wild in northern California, southern Oregon, and Colorado, St. John's wort has been used as medicine for more than 2,400 years. To date, no evidence exists that taking the two herbs causes side effects; in fact, they complement each other quite nicely.

CHAPTER 4

The Heart of the Matter

The heart . . . a symbol of courage, of love, of life, of morality. Indeed, no other organ of the body carries as much emotional and psychological weight as the human heart. In every culture, from the ashrams of India to the modern operating rooms of the United States, the heart is recognized as a vital, precious source of life and vitality. Traditional Chinese medicine calls the heart the Emperor of the organs and *The Internal Medicine Classic,* an ancient TCM textbook, states: "The heart commands all of the organs and viscera, houses the spirit, and controls the emotions. In Chinese, the word for heart (*shen*) is also used to denote 'mind.' "

Physiologically, and in both the East and the West, the heart lies at the center of a vast network of vessels that control the circulation and distribution of blood, and therefore all other organs depend on it for sustenance. Just for a moment, consider that

- Each beat of your heart transports oxygen and nutrients to more than 300 trillion cells throughout the body.

- Every day, the average heart beats 100,000 times, so that if you live to be seventy years old, your heart will beat about 2.5 billion times.
- The heart beats approximately once every second, sending about five quarts of blood coursing through the circulatory system every minute.
- In total area, the capillary walls are equal to about 60,000 to 70,000 square feet, or roughly the area of one and a half football fields.

Keeping these statistics in mind, consider how most of us take for granted how hard and how well our cardiovascular systems work—as long as we keep them healthy. And there's the rub: Cardiovascular disease remains the nation's number-one killer; in 1994, for example, it claimed the lives of more than 950,000 people, representing 41.8 percent of all deaths in this country that year. Although there is a genetic—and thus unpreventable—component to cardiovascular disease, most causes of heart attack, stroke, peripheral vascular disease, and other related conditions remain under your control to prevent. Taking ginkgo biloba extract is one of the ways you can help to significantly reduce your risks of developing cardiovascular disease.

In Chapter 2, you learned a little bit about how your heart and the vast system of blood vessels work together to bring oxygen and vital nutrients to every cell of the body, and to take away waste products before they collect in and among the tissues. We also described some of the reasons why blood flow and heart function can become blocked or disturbed, as well as how ginkgo biloba works to keep such blockages from occurring. Here we'll explore that subject in more depth, starting with a description of the main risk factors for cardiovascular disease.

RISK FACTORS FOR CARDIOVASCULAR DISEASE

Cardiovascular disease is a blanket term that encompasses a wide variety of related conditions. Some involve problems with the vessels themselves, others with the heart, and still others with blood components like platelets and red blood cells. Often, a problem in one area of the system has widespread effects. At the heart of most cases of cardiovascular disease is the process we described in Chapter 2: arteriosclerosis, or the narrowing and hardening of arteries with plaque—fatty deposits of cholesterol and, often, blood clots. Arteriosclerosis can result in blood loss to vital tissues. When this occurs to the heart muscle itself, angina (chest pain) or even death of heart tissue (myocardial infarction) may result. When it occurs in the brain, a "brain attack," also called a cerebrovascular event or stroke, may result. Blood loss to the legs results in a condition called peripheral vascular disease and painful symptoms known as intermittent claudication.

When it comes to these three main groups of cardiovascular disease, the risk factors—those conditions or habits that make it more likely that you'll develop them—are quite similar, if not identical. In all but a few uncontrollable risk factors, such as your age, gender, and family history, taking ginkgo biloba extract—especially in combination with other medical, nutritional, and lifestyle modifications—can help alleviate or offset the risks. We'll discuss ginkgo biloba's role in cardiovascular disease and treatment later in the Chapter. In the meantime, here are the risk factors most commonly related to cardiovascular disease:

- *Age.* Your risk of cardiovascular disease increases as you get older. More than half of those who have heart attacks are 65 years of age or older, and four out of five of those who die of such attacks are over age 65. On the other hand, a full 5 percent of heart attacks occur in people under age 40, and 28 percent of stroke victims are under the age of 65.
- *Gender.* At all ages, men are at more risk for cardiovascular disease than are women. After menopause (and the loss of protection from the female hormone estrogen), however, women's rates quickly rise to nearly those of men. Both heart attacks and strokes are more deadly in women than in men, both because women are often unaware of the high risk they have of developing cardiovascular disease and because the symptoms of heart attack tend to be more subtle in women than in men.
- *Family history.* There is no question that some people have a significantly greater likelihood of having cardiovascular disease because they inherit a tendency to do so from their parents. In most cases, the specific way in which inheritance plays a role is unclear. However, even someone with a family history can dramatically reduce his or her risks by controlling other risk factors.
- *High blood pressure.* Also known as hypertension, high blood pressure is the risk factor for cardiovascular disease that affects the greatest number of Americans. Estimates vary, but anywhere from 35 million to more than 60 million people have elevated blood pressure. One way that high blood pressure damages blood vessels is by increasing the inflammatory response, which, as you may remember from Chapter 2, brings harmful chemicals to the cell linings of blood vessels, weakening them

and making them more susceptible to plaque buildup and arteriosclerosis. Hypertension often occurs together with other risk factors, particularly obesity, elevated levels of cholesterol and triglycerides, and diabetes mellitus.

Chronic, untreated high blood pressure is an important risk factor in heart disease, stroke, and peripheral vascular disease. In addition, recent research published in the American Heart Association journal *Stroke* indicates that high blood pressure speeds the loss of memory and other cognitive abilities in the elderly, and actually causes their brain to shrink in size—and this problem occurs even in the absence of stroke.

• *High cholesterol.* Having too much of certain kinds of fats and other lipids puts you at higher risk of developing plaques that narrow the blood vessels and reduce blood flow to vital areas of the body (arteriosclerosis). Cholesterol is a lipid essential for a number of vital processes, including nerve function, cell repair and reproduction, and the formation of various hormones. The body, however, manufactures all the cholesterol it needs, so that any cholesterol you consume is extra and can lead to health problems.

Cholesterol travels through the bloodstream by combining with other lipids and certain proteins. When combined, these substances are called lipoproteins. One type of lipoprotein, called high-density lipoprotein (HDL), is beneficial to the body because it carries cholesterol away from blood vessel walls. Another type of lipoprotein, low-density lipoprotein (LDL), is considered harmful because it carries about two-thirds of circulating cholesterol to the cells. Research indicates that LDL cholesterol may become harmful only after it has been oxidized, or combined with oxygen. Oxidation occurs primarily when the cells become damaged by free radicals, unstable molecules that enter the body through the food you eat and the air you breathe.

- *High homocysteine levels.* Current research indicates that cholesterol is not the only—or even the most important—culprit when it comes to cardiovascular disease. In fact, a quarter of heart attacks occur in people without elevated cholesterol or other known risk factors. Homocysteine, an amino acid found in the blood, plays an important role as well. People with homocysteine levels in the top 5 percent of normal have been shown to have three times the risk of a heart attack than those with levels in the lower 90 percent. Currently, the only available treatment for this condition is taking vitamin B_6 and folic acid—two powerful antioxidants. B vitamins are involved in many cellular processes.

- *Smoking.* A smoker's risk of cardiovascular disease is more than twice that of a nonsmoker. Overall, experts estimate that 30 to 40 percent of the approximately 500,000 deaths from coronary artery disease each year can be attributed to smoking. The nicotine in cigarette smoke increases heart and vessel activity, while many of the other toxic substances contribute to the acceleration of arteriosclerosis. Cigarette smoke raises the amount of fat and cholesterol circulating in the bloodstream, which form plaque on artery walls. Carbon monoxide, another ingredient in cigarette smoke, damages the cells that form the inner linings of arterial walls, making them more susceptible to plaque buildup.

To make matters worse, carbon monoxide is carried through the bloodstream by the same blood component—hemoglobin—that transports oxygen. The more carbon monoxide in the bloodstream, then, the less oxygen is being carried to the vital organs, including the heart and brain. Therefore, at the same time that nicotine is stimulating heart and blood vessel activity, carbon monoxide prevents oxygen from helping the body do this extra work. Over time, this extra stress weakens both heart and vessel walls and further paves the way for arteriosclerosis and hemorrhage. Finally, cigarette smoke also causes chemical changes in the blood itself, causing it to become more viscous, or sticky, which results in the formation of large blood clots.

- *Diabetes mellitus.* Defined as an inability to properly metabolize carbohydrates, diabetes mellitus also represents a significant risk for cardiovascular disease. Experts feel this is due in part to the fact that people with diabetes have much higher levels of fat in the bloodstream than do those with healthy blood sugar metabolism.

  In many cases, the problem is that insulin levels become elevated in response to certain carbohydrates, particularly grains and potatoes. These foods are said to have a high "glycemic index," and the resulting elevated insulin levels make weight loss difficult as well as increase inflammation and platelet thickening. This insulin is particularly damaging to arterial walls and leads to increased cardiac risk. In addition, both the small and large blood vessels of those with diabetes tend to thicken abnormally, conditions known as microangiopathy and macroangiopathy. Diabetes also may trigger the development of high blood pressure and arteriosclerosis. Diets that emphasize protein and low glycemic-index carbohydrates like vegetables are used to combat this hyperinsulinism.

- *Obesity.* Being more than 20 percent over your ideal weight is a known risk factor for cardiovascular disease of all types. Even 10 extra pounds places a burden on the heart and blood vessels; for each pound of excess weight, the heart is forced to pump blood through an additional 700 miles of blood vessels a day. Overweight people also tend to eat too much fat and cholesterol, which contribute to the development of arteriosclerosis. Obesity and diabetes are twin threats; most people with diabetes are overweight and many overweight individuals will develop diabetes. The combination of hypertension, diabetes, and obesity often leads to heart attack and stroke.

- *Sedentary lifestyle.* It's been official since 1992: The American Heart Association now designates inactivity as one of the four top risk factors for the development of cardiovascular disease. The Centers for Disease Control in Atlanta, Georgia, estimate that about 250,000 deaths per year can be attributed to a sedentary lifestyle.

- *Stress.* Although there still isn't a proper definition for what we mean by harmful stress, there remains little doubt of a connection between unrelieved high stress and cardiovascular disease. In a recent study, for instance, performed at Duke University and published in the February 1998 issue of *New Choices: Living Even Better After 50,* stress caused a threefold higher risk of a heart attack and death in men and women with ischemia, or reduced blood flow to the heart.

Chronic stress causes blood pressure and heart rate levels to remain elevated. High levels of the stress hormone cortisol may lead to elevated blood sugar, platelet stickiness, and, some research shows, an increased level of blood cholesterol. All of the stress hormones have a tendency to increase free-radical formation, which can lead to the oxidation of cholesterol, forming the "bad" cholesterol that damages and clogs blood vessels. Finally, chronic muscle tension can deplete the body's store of magnesium and potassium, creating an excess of calcium and sodium. The latter two minerals may act to cause vasospasm—abnormal constriction of the arteries, including the coronary arteries, which may result in a heart attack.

- *Poor diet.* A diet high in fat and refined carbohydrates, particularly white flour products and sugar, and low in antioxidants (the free radical–fighting substances contained in many fresh fruits and vegetables) contributes to the development and acceleration of cardiovascular disease.

As you can see, many of the risk factors for cardiovascular disease are under your power to control, and we'll give you some tips on how to do just that—including information on the benefits of taking ginkgo biloba extract—later in the chapter. Now let's take a closer look at the three most common cardiovascular problems: heart disease, stroke, and peripheral vascular disease.

HEART DISEASE/HEART ATTACK

In 1997, a survey performed by the Quaker Oats Company revealed a shocking statistic: Despite decades of a massive education effort by the U.S. government and private organizations, more than half of Americans still do not realize that heart disease is the leading cause of death in the United States. According to the survey, 57 percent named other sources, including 28 percent who thought cancer was the leading cause of death. Yet, according to statistics compiled by the Centers for Disease Control, almost one in two Americans die of cardiovascular disease, 500,000 of them of heart attacks. The large majority of heart attacks result from coronary artery disease.

The Heart in Action

The heart, a fist-size muscular pump, has four chambers, the left and right atria on top, and the right and left ventricles on the bottom. It also has four valves, each with its own set of flaps that open and close as your heart expands or contracts, allowing a stable flow of blood through the heart. These four chambers beat in a precise manner, controlled by electrical impulses that originate in the sinus node, a cluster of cells located in the right atrium. Although the sinus node usually produces electrical impulses in a steady, predictable rate, this rate can sometimes alter according to emotional or hormonal changes (your heart rate may rise when you become worried or upset, for example, or race or skip a beat due to the hormonal changes that occur during pregnancy).

Surrounding the heart like a crown (or corona, for which it is named) are the two coronary arteries. The left main coronary artery branches off the main vessel (the aorta) and divides in two. The right coronary artery comes off the aorta and supplies blood to the right and bottom parts of the heart. Although the body's entire volume of blood passes through the heart's chambers every minute, only about 5 percent of the total amount is available for the heart's own needs. The coronary arteries, which are only an eighth to a fifth of an inch in diameter, are the sole conduits for the supply of blood to the heart. Without adequate blood flow to the heart muscle, the heart itself is unable to function properly.

Oxygen Deprivation (Ischemia) and Heart Attack

For the majority of people suffering from coronary artery disease, the supply of oxygenated blood is reduced due to arteriosclerosis—a progressive narrowing of the open channels of the coronary arteries. As we've discussed, the buildup of plaque is a gradual process, and it may take 20 years or more before the arteries are blocked enough to produce symptoms such as shortness of breath and chest pain. If the blockage is total, a heart attack may result.

A primary symptom of coronary artery disease is chest pain, or angina. Angina is not itself a disease but a symptom, usually of oxygen deprivation due to arteriosclerosis, a condition also known as ischemia. People who suffer from angina describe a feeling of discomfort or pain, often using such words as "pressure" or "heaviness." This pain is usually located in the center of the chest but may radiate to or occur only in the neck, shoulder, arm, or lower jaw. For most people, the pain almost always occurs during or after physical activity and/or emotional stress. Ischemia may occasionally occur without symptoms of angina or other discomfort, which earns it the name "silent ischemia." Angina is a sign that a more serious problem—a heart attack—may be developing.

Heart attacks, also known as acute myocardial infarction, are frequently the result of coronary artery disease. A blood clot or muscular spasm in a narrowed coronary vessel may suddenly block it completely, triggering an infarction (death of tissue) in the area of the heart muscle that is normally nourished by that artery. Another common cause of heart attacks is sudden spasm of a coronary artery, triggered by emotional or physical stress. A heart attack can be dangerous, because irreparable heart damage may develop within a short time after the muscle is deprived of oxygen.

The more quickly treatment begins after the onset of a heart attack, the less severe the injury to the muscle is likely to be. The symptoms of a heart attack include:

- Uncomfortable pressure, fullness, squeezing, or pain in the center of the chest, lasting two minutes or longer
- Pain spreading to the shoulders, neck, or arms
- Light-headedness, fainting, sweating, nausea, or shortness of breath

Later, we'll describe some of the most common and effective treatments for heart disease and heart attacks. Right now, let's look at what happens when the blockage of blood vessels occurs in another vital organ: the brain.

STROKE

In February 1998, the American Heart Association announced that the official estimate of the number of Americans afflicted with a stroke each year—500,000—is too low, that at least 731,000 people are struck by "brain attacks" every year, either their first or a recurrent episode. Stroke, also referred to as a cerebrovascular accident or CVA, is a disturbance in brain function—sometimes permanent—caused by either a blockage or a rupture in a vessel supplying blood to the brain.

As discussed in Chapter 3, in order to function properly, nerve cells within the brain must have a continuous supply of blood, oxygen, and glucose (blood sugar). If this supply is impaired, parts of the brain may stop functioning temporarily. If the impairment is severe, or lasts long enough, brain cells die and permanent damage follows. There are two main types of stroke: hemorrhagic strokes, which account for about 20 to 25 percent of all strokes, and ischemic strokes, which account for about 70 percent of strokes. Hemorrhagic strokes involve blood seeping from a hole in a blood vessel wall into either the brain itself or the space around the brain. Most people who have hemorrhagic strokes have a history of hypertension, diabetes, and arteriosclerosis. Ischemic strokes are caused by a lack of blood flow to the brain. In some cases, oxygen deprivation is caused by a clot (thrombus) that blocks blood flow in an artery. Another kind of ischemic stroke involving a clot is called a cerebral embolism, which is caused by a wandering clot that forms in one part of the body, breaks loose, and travels in the bloodstream until it lodges in an artery in the brain or in a vessel leading to the brain. A third form is called lacunar infarctions, which are the result of the complete blockage of arterioles, the very small ends of the arteries that penetrate deep into the brain.

PERIPHERAL VASCULAR DISEASE

Peripheral vascular disease (PVD) is essentially the same condition as coronary artery disease, which it often accompanies, and occurs in the same way as stroke. In all three conditions, plaque deposits form in arteries, decreasing their blood-carrying capacity. That causes pain during exertion because the muscles served by the clogged arteries aren't getting enough oxygen. While the pain this blockage causes is called angina when it occurs in the heart, it is called claudication when it occurs in the legs.

Peripheral vascular disease is the leading cause of amputations in this country. It generally strikes those over the age of 45 and is a frequent complication of diabetes. As is true for other forms of cardiovascular disease, PVD is more likely to affect smokers, people with high blood pressure and/or high cholesterol levels, those with a family history of artery disease, and those who are obese.

A 10-year study at the University of California reported a high death rate from cardiovascular disease among patients with even mild peripheral artery blockage. For patients with severe leg artery problems, the 10-year mortality rate was as much as 15 times that of people with no PVD.

The symptom of PVD is cramping pain in the muscles of the calves, thighs, or hips during exercise. At first, the pain goes away quickly when you stop exercising. But, as the disease progresses, the pain begins earlier during exertion and becomes more severe. When the tissues become chronically starved for blood, you may experience foot pains while at rest that are worse when you elevate the foot. In its advanced stages, leg ulcers, even gangrene, can set in. A particularly severe form of

PVD affects cigarette smokers almost exclusively. Called Buerger's disease, it leads to marked decreases in peripheral circulation, often leading to amputation.

It should be noted that not all cases of decreased peripheral circulation are caused by arteriosclerosis. Raynaud's disease, for instance, is a relatively rare condition, seen most commonly in women between the ages of 15 and 50. It is caused by an overconstriction of blood vessels in fingers, toes, and, less frequently, the ears and nose. The cause of the condition is unknown.

TREATMENT AND PREVENTION STRATEGIES

Needless to say, the damage that results from a lack of blood flow to the brain, the heart, or the extremities can result in severe disability and even death. It goes far beyond the scope of this book to offer a complete description of the complex diagnostic and treatment strategies available to help those who have had a stroke or heart attack. Every day, new medications and surgical techniques are developed that help more and more people survive and thrive after a cardiovascular event. If you want to know more about heart attack and stroke and what happens when they occur, please see the list of books and Internet Web sites we've collected in the Resources section at the end of the book.

In the meantime, let's work at helping you *prevent* these conditions from ever developing in the first place. Certainly, when it comes to cardiovascular disease, prevention is the very best medicine.

Ginkgo Biloba and Your Cardiovascular System

First, before we go any further, DO NOT start taking ginkgo biloba extract if you are taking any medication for cardiovascular disease that acts to thin the blood—and that includes prescription medication like Coumadin and the over-the-counter wonder drug called aspirin (unless you talk to your doctor first). As we'll discuss in Chapter 9, blood thinners and anticoagulants are among the only drugs counterindicated with GBE—taking them together could result in excess bleeding.

That said, as long as you're not taking an anticoagulant, GBE can help prevent the development of cardiovascular disease and mitigate the effects of disease that are already present for most people. Take a look back at the risk factors for cardiovascular disease. Apart from your family history, gender, and age, which you cannot change, your risks all involve disease processes that ginkgo biloba can help to prevent or at least slow down. Indeed, a 1992 German study reported in the journal *Arzneimittel-Forschung* provided evidence that GBE, taken over a long period, can reduce cardiovascular problems, including heart disease, stroke, peripheral vascular disease, high blood pressure, excess cholesterol, and diabetes. Let's see how GBE affects the cardiovascular system by looking at the risk factors one by one:

- *High blood pressure.* GBE can help counter the damage to the vessel walls caused by chronic, untreated hypertension by preventing or reducing the release of platelet-activating factor (PAF). As you may remember, this substance increases the stickiness of the blood and thus contributes to the process of arteriosclerosis. GBE also helps maintain the integrity and elasticity of vessels, which may help to reduce high blood pressure in another way.

- *High cholesterol level.* Since cholesterol may become harmful only after being oxidized by free radicals, GBE's powerful antioxidant effects may help counter this process and thus mitigate another major risk factor for cardiovascular disease.
- *High homocysteine level.* Once again, GBE's antioxidant properties may help to reduce the levels of this apparently harmful amino acid. Currently, the only treatment available for high homocysteine levels involves the use of vitamin B_6 and folic acid. More than likely, GBE will be added to that list.
- *Cigarette smoking.* Although nothing can undo the damage done by smoking—except quitting as soon as possible—it may be that GBE can help protect your cardiovascular system from some of the damage done by the nicotine and other toxins you inhale every time you puff on a cigarette. For instance, GBE helps reduce the stickiness of platelets (which cigarette smoke triggers) and reduces the tendency of blood vessels to spasm.
- *Diabetes mellitus.* Controlling your blood sugar by monitoring your diet and modifying your exercise habits is clearly the best way to prevent diabetes from affecting your cardiovascular system. Taking GBE may help, however, since it may be able to protect the blood vessel linings from becoming damaged by high levels of circulating blood sugar and insulin.
- *Stress.* One of the side effects of stress is vasospasm—the sudden contraction and constriction of blood vessels. GBE helps alleviate this tendency, and also counteracts the effects of stress hormones

on blood platelet stickiness, thereby slowing down the arteriosclerotic process.

Furthermore, several studies show the effect GBE has on specific cardiovascular challenges. In 1995, for instance, a Chinese animal study reported that the free radical–scavenging properties of GBE might be helpful to the heart. For the experiment, researchers injected the coronary arteries of one group of rabbits suffering from oxygen deprivation with GBE and those of another group with a saline solution. The heart tissue of those given GBE was less swollen and torn than was the heart tissues of those given the saline. These results, reported in *Biochemistry and Biology International* in January 1995, suggest that the antioxidant properties of ginkgo biloba protect the heart, while ginkgo's ability to help the blood heal damaged tissues helps the heart resist damage.

When it comes to peripheral vascular disease and its primary painful symptom, intermittent claudication, GBE's effects have been proved in several studies. In nine double-blind, randomized clinical trials of GBE versus placebo in two matched groups of people with peripheral vascular disease, GBE was shown to be quite active and superior to placebo. Not only were pain-free walking distances dramatically increased, but clinical observation showed an increased blood flow through the affected limbs.

Aspirin and Your Heart

Although aspirin cannot prevent cardiovascular disease—anymore than ginkgo biloba can, for that matter—this remarkable substance appears to have significant beneficial effects on the heart, vessels, and blood. A study at Harvard University found that for selected patients, one aspirin taken every other day reduced heart attack risk by 50 percent. And, when taken during or immediately following a heart attack, aspirin appears to significantly reduce the risk of death during the first five weeks after the attack.

Aspirin works to prevent heart attacks (and perhaps stroke and peripheral vascular disease, though these conditions are less well studied in relation to aspirin) by thinning the blood and making it less likely to clot. In that way, aspirin is similar to GBE. However, unlike GBE, aspirin can have significant side effects, including excess bleeding and stomach irritation. The American Heart Association recommends that you talk to your doctor before deciding to take regular doses of aspirin to prevent a heart attack or other forms of cardiovascular disease.

Eating Right

Again, providing a complete dietary prescription for a healthy heart goes far beyond the scope of this book—and you'll read more about healthy eating in Chapter 8. In the meantime, we thought we'd offer you a look at the new dietary recommendations developed to reduce hypertension, one of the most important—and common—risk factors for cardiovascular disease. The diet prescribed is one that offers a wide variety of foods, in moderate amounts, and thus appears to be fairly easy to manage and enjoyable.

A study published in the April 1997 issue of the *New England Journal of Medicine* proved what experts had suspected for quite some time: Eating a diet rich in fresh fruits and vegetables and low-fat dairy products will indeed reduce your risk of developing cardiovascular disease. People who ate nine to 10 daily servings of fruits and vegetables (about twice the usual amount in Americans' diets) and three daily servings of low-fat dairy products (again, about double the amount in most Americans' diets) lowered their blood pressures as much as any one prescription antihypertension medication did. Fruits and vegetables contain flavonoids and other free radical–fighting substances, which helps to explain this remarkable connection.

The diet researchers used in this study, called the DASH diet, was used primarily to reduce hypertension. Here's how many servings of what kinds of food were in the DASH diet's 2,000-calorie-a-day regimen:

- 7 to 8 servings of grain or grain products
- 4 to 5 vegetables a day
- 4 to 5 fruits a day
- 2 to 3 servings of low-fat or nonfat dairy products
- 2 or fewer servings of meat, poultry, or fish
- 4 to 5 servings *per week,* of nuts, seeds, and beans
- 2 to 3 tsps. a day of oil or other fats

In addition to eating plenty of fresh fruits and vegetables (and thus the powerful antioxidants and other substances they contain), you also may want to increase your intake of dietary fiber. An increase in daily soluble fiber intake by just 3 grams reduced the risk of coronary death by 27 percent. Whole-grain breads made from rye, oats, barley, and wheat are perfect sources of dietary fiber, as is oatmeal. According to studies published in the December issue of *Circulation* and *The American Journal of Clinical Nutrition,* eating more oat soluble fiber improves health and may extend longevity by reducing levels of blood glucose, insulin, and triglycerides. It turns out that eating oatmeal for breakfast in the morning may be especially helpful. However, it appears that to attain these benefits, you have to use whole oats and cook them slowly. Neither quick-cook or instant oatmeal has the same effect. The *Circulation* study showed that oats have twice as much beta-glucan—a type of soluble fiber—than rye, barley, or wheat. You can get 3 grams of oat soluble fiber in 1½ cups of cooked oatmeal.

Antioxidants: Whole Foods and Supplements

Certain vitamins, particularly vitamins C and E, beta-carotene, and the minerals selenium and zinc, may be helpful in preventing heart disease. What do these vitamins do to help keep the cardiovascular system so healthy? In addition to scavenging free radicals, most antioxidants also help reduce platelet stickiness, aid in the breakdown of fats, help lower blood cholesterol levels, and increase the effectiveness of certain enzymes in the body.

One study on the role of antioxidants on heart disease was performed by Joann Manson, M.D., and Charles Hennekens, M.D., of Harvard Medical School and Brigham and Women's Hospital in Boston. After monitoring the diet and vitamin use of 87,000 nurses for more than a decade, the investigators found that the women whose vitamin E consumption was in the upper 20 percent had a 35 percent lower risk of heart disease—even when all other factors, like smoking, blood pressure, and cholesterol levels, were taken into account. Those whose beta-carotene consumption was in the upper 20 percent had a 22 percent lower risk of heart disease.

According to a study in the American Heart Association journal *Circulation,* as much as one-fifth of the

U.S. population may be at increased risk of heart attacks and stroke because they do not eat enough food with vitamin B_6 and folic acid. Those in the study with a B_6 deficiency were almost twice as likely to have heart disease and stroke than were those without a deficiency. Again, the association of these two substances with heart disease may be connected to their effects on homocysteine, the amino acid known to damage the lining of blood vessels. Low levels of vitamin B_6 can lead to elevations in homocysteine. Talk to your doctor and see the Resources list in this book if you're interested in exploring the use of vitamins and minerals in your quest for cardiovascular health.

Other ways you can reduce your risk of heart disease, stroke, peripheral vascular disease, and other forms of cardiovascular disease include the following:

- *Lose weight.* Obesity is a major risk factor for cardiovascular disease of all types, and as many as 40 percent of all Americans are obese. Although losing weight—and keeping it off—can be very difficult, it is essential. If you want to maintain your health, you've got to maintain a healthy weight. The best way to diet, all experts agree, is to eat relatively small portions of a wide variety of foods—and to exercise!

- *Keep it moving.* The purely physical benefits of exercise are almost too many to list: Your heart will be able to pump more blood and your vessels will be able to deliver more oxygen to the cells throughout the body in a more efficient manner. Over time, blood cholesterol levels are reduced and the ratio of "bad cholesterol" to "good cholesterol" is decreased. Over the long haul, exercise also reduces blood pressure and increases blood flow into the smallest arteries and veins, thus ensuring that every cell in the body receives proper nutrition. In addition, exercise has significant psychological and emotional benefits. People who exercise find that they not only feel better physically but also have a renewed sense of emotional well-being both during and in between exercise sessions. Again, we'll discuss how to make exercise a part of your life in Chapter 8.

- *Stop smoking.* Experts now recognize that nicotine is every bit as addictive as other narcotics, and therefore extremely difficult to give up. Fortunately, there's help out there if you need it. Contact the American Heart Association, the American Lung Association, and even your local YWCA for information about stop-smoking groups in your area. You can also talk to your doctor or nutritionist about natural substances, like chlorophyll and the amino acid l-glutamine, that may help you beat the habit.

Unfortunately, the people who need to stop smoking the most are the least likely to stop, says a new Mayo Clinic study of heart patients published in the March 1998 issue of *Mayo Clinic Proceedings.* Mayo researchers looked at the smoking patterns of more than 5,400 patients who had angioplasties (vessel-clearing procedures) over a 16-year period. Of this group, 63 percent continued to smoke after their procedure, 51 percent continued to smoke even after a prior heart attack, and less than 10 percent sought help from a Mayo Clinic Nicotine Dependence Center. The study found that patients most likely to continue smoking were those who would benefit most by quitting—that is,

younger patients who smoked the most and had
more risk factors for cardiovascular disease.

- *Reduce stress.* Your heart and blood vessels take it
the hardest when you're under constant stress and
tension: Raising the blood pressure and heart rate is
an essential part of the fight-or-flight response. In
Chapter 8, we'll describe some of the most effective
stress-reduction methods available, including meditation, progressive relaxation, and even biofeedback. And it's important to understand that stress
comes in all forms—depression as well as anxiety
can be disruptive to the health of your cardiovascular system, though for different reasons. According
to a study presented by Johns Hopkins researchers
at the American Heart Association's 1997 70th Annual Scientific Sessions, nearly one in four people
suffer from depression after a heart attack—and
these people are less likely to comply with their
doctors' advice to modify their diets and exercise
habits.

Now that you've read about your heart and circulation, it's time to move on to another system of the
body: the immune system and the allergic response.

Find Out More About . . .

. . . Ginkgo Biloba Extract

Q. Because heart disease runs in my family, I'm currently taking half an aspirin a day, and no other medication. Could I
also take GBE?

A. You probably can take a small amount of aspirin with GBE

and experience no ill effects. However, talk to your doctor before doing so, as both substances are blood thinners. Because GBE doesn't irritate the stomach lining in most people, you may want to cut out your use of aspirin and replace it with GBE.

. . . Raynaud's Disease

Q. I suffer from Raynaud's disease. How should I treat it?

A. That depends on the cause. If your doctor tells you that arteriosclerosis has blocked the arteries leading to your legs, there may be new treatment to help you. Called VasoCare, this treatment is a cellular therapy in which cells from a patient's own blood are modified in special ways and then injected back into the body. Research indicates that VasoCare therapy benefits patients in two ways: by improving the function of blood vessel linings to control blood flow, and by reducing autoimmunity—or the inflammatory process that occurs when blood cells are damaged by high blood pressure and immune system cells rush to the area.

. . . Eating Right

Q. What about drinking wine? I've heard different things about it. Is it good for your heart?

A. A fascinating study in an August 1997 issue of the *American Journal of Cardiology* showed that moderate wine and alcohol consumption does play a role in preventing coronary heart disease and, presumably, other forms of cardiovascular disease. The study also showed that wine appeared to be most protective for women, while beer appeared to be most protective in men. Other studies indicate that wine does have advantages over other forms of alcohol. Wine has phenolic compounds, which reduce the rate of LDL oxidation, platelet formation, and the buildup of fat in the arteries. The Copenhagen City Heart Study in 1995 found distinct overall mortality advantages for wine drinkers compared to drinkers of other beverages.

Q. I've heard that eating fish is a good way to cut your risk of developing cardiovascular disease. What's the connection?

A. A report issued at the American Heart Association's 70th Scientific Sessions found that eating a lot of fish—even more than a strict vegetarian diet—lowers certain kinds of harmful lipids in the bloodstream, thereby lowering the risk of a heart attack. Scientists believe that omega-3 fatty acids, contained in fish oil, protect against arteriosclerosis by altering cholesterol metabolism.

Losing Weight . . .

Q. What does BMI mean, and how do you measure it?

A. Researchers have used body mass index, or BMI, as a way to assess obesity in large populations and in scientific studies. Since recommendations from major organizations like the American Heart Association and American Cancer Society use BMI rather than pounds, it's important to understand what these numbers mean and why they are important for good health.

BMI is simply a mathematical calculation that determines your weight-to-height ratio. You can find your BMI with a simple formula:

1. Multiply your weight in pounds by 705.
2. Divide the result by your height in inches.
3. Divide that result by your height in inches again, and you've got your BMI.

For optimal health, your BMI should fall between 18.5 and 25 throughout your life. Your risk of developing cardiovascular disease, and other health problems, rises the higher your BMI.

CHAPTER 5

Taming the Inflammatory Response

Out with the carbon dioxide, in with the oxygen. Every day, most people perform the simple, unremarkable act of breathing thousands of times without giving it a second thought. Most people also manage to make it through their days without breaking out into a rash, or rubbing their irritated eyes, or sneezing uncontrollably. On the other hand, there is a significant and not so silent majority of men, women, and children who struggle to take easy breaths and exist in the environment without irritation and pain—namely, the 46 million who suffer from asthma and allergies.

Jose is one of those people, having suffered since childhood with debilitating symptoms of allergies to a variety of substances including pollen, dust mites, and cat dander. Tired of taking antihistamines and bronchodilators—two conventional medications—on a nearly constant basis, he decided to visit a holistic practitioner for some advice on treating his condition more naturally. In addition to making changes in his diet and helping identify (and then avoid) the triggers of his allergic reactions, Jose's doctor prescribed ginkgo biloba extract. Since Jose's been taking ginkgo and following his new diet, his symptoms have stabilized and he needs to use conventional medication only on an occasional basis.

Asthma and allergies, which affect the respiratory system and the immune system, were among the first conditions to be treated with ginkgo biloba. In fact, the first Chinese medical text, published in 2,800 B.C., the MATERIA MEDICA, describes using ginkgo to treat chronic coughing and congestion. Chinese practitioners considered the herb to be a lung astringent and a tonic for a weakened condition. Today, traditional Chinese doctors continue to prescribe ginkgo to treat respiratory illnesses related to allergies, just as Western scientists are exploring its use for these conditions, too.

What makes ginkgo so effective when it comes to allergies and respiratory problems? We'll discuss that in more depth later in the chapter. Before we do that, however, it's important for you to gain an understanding of the allergic response and the way it can affect the body.

IMMUNITY OUT OF CONTROL

The healthy human body is a virtual citadel—a self-contained structure that protects itself against harmful invaders from the outside world. It has a massive defense system that starts with a protective wall (the skin), a first line of defense (the tiny hairs of the nose, certain enzymes in saliva), and a complex and organized army of cells patrolling the internal environment. When functioning as it should, this defense organization allows the body's population of organs, tissues, and fluids to flourish. Constantly streaming through lymph and blood vessels, immune cells attempt to ensure that outside enemies do not upset the balance within.

The immune system's special characteristic is the ability to recognize other cells in the body. It can tell the difference between harmful microbes, cancer cells, and the body's own healthy cells. Put very simply, it's as if each cell wears a uniform and the patrolling guards—white blood cells called lymphocytes—can distinguish one uniform from another, friend or foe.

When a cell provokes a response from the immune system—when lymphocytes recognize an enemy "uniform"—that cell is called an antigen. Viruses, bacteria, protozoa, and fungi are antigens because they provoke an immune system response once they enter the body. Transplanted tissues and organs, and sometimes our own cells (if they are cancer cells), are also antigens, because lymphocytes recognize them as enemies and begin a process of defense against them. This type of immune response is called auto-immunity.

In essence, a "misfiring" of this defense system causes an allergy. For reasons as yet poorly understood, immune system cells mistakenly identify harmless substances—like cat dander or pollen—as antigens and mount an attack against them. When harmless antigens cause an immune system response, the antigens are called "allergens." The symptoms of allergies, including wheezing (asthma), sneezing, and skin rashes, represents the outward signs of your body's attempt to rid itself of what it perceives to be harmful enemies.

Today, the body must protect itself from a greater and greater number of potential foes. We must guard not only against the natural organisms—viruses, bacteria, fungi—that have always been present, but also against a whole host of synthetic pollutants in the air, soil, food, and even in the medicines we take. Many scientists believe that so many people suffer from allergies and asthma today because the sheer number of substances—harmful and good—entering our bodies everyday simply overwhelms the immune system. The "soldiers" in charge of the body's defense become hypervigilant, "trigger-happy," so to speak.

Immune System Soldiers

Two main classes of immune system soldiers protect the body, T cells and B cells, each of which responds in a different way to threats from potential enemies. T cells have a molecular code on their surface that directly responds to specific antigens, which means that T cells can destroy enemy cells on contact. T cells also work with other immune system cells to either stimulate activity or suppress immune function.

B cells, on the other hand, do not kill antigens directly, but instead produce a type of immune system cell called an antibody or immunoglobulin. Antibodies are the primary defense cells against most types of antigens. The body produces them when a B cell comes into contact with an antigen that it recognizes as an enemy. Once the antigen locks onto the B cell, the B cell rapidly and repeatedly divides, creating hundreds of new cells (called plasma cells) that release antibodies in massive amounts.

Antibodies attempt to render antigens harmless in a number of ways. If the antigen produces a toxin, for instance, the antibody may be able to directly neutralize the harmful substance. Or antibodies can force enemy microbes together into a clump, allowing other immune system cells to rapidly destroy them.

Once the crisis that stimulated their release is over, antibodies circulate in the body for some time, then die off. At the same time that activated B cells produce antibodies, however, they also produce what are called "memory cells." As their name implies, memory cells immediately recognize the specific antigen that first provoked their production—whether it's a cold virus or an allergen like a sprig of pollen. When that antigen enters the body, memory cells quickly stimulate an immune system reaction. That's why it sometimes takes only moments after you come into contact with an allergen for your eyes to start to water or your bronchial tubes to constrict.

Antibodies are also known as immunoglobulins, or Igs. Scientists have identified five major classes of immunoglobulins, each of which acts in a slightly different way against foreign invaders. IgG immunoglobulins, for instance, fight infection from bacteria, fungi, and viruses. They also appear to be involved in certain allergic responses, including food allergies.

It is the IgE immunoglobulins that are most involved in allergic reactions. Concentrated in the lung, the skin, and the cells of mucous membranes, they offer the body its prime protection against antigens from the environment. IgE molecules (and other immunoglobulins) react to otherwise benign substances like pollen, cat dander, and certain foods and chemicals, among others. They act aggressively to rid the body of the offending allergens and, by doing so, create irritating and sometimes painful—even deadly—symptoms and reactions. In people with allergies, the IgE antibodies to their specific allergens exist by the millions.

When antibodies encounter their specific allergen, they immediately trigger the release of certain immune system cells, including the compound PAF (platelet-activating factor). PAF activates several kinds of immune cells, including neutrophils, eosinophils, macrophages, and endothelial cells—all of which secrete chemicals that create inflammation. As you may remember from Chapter 2, the inflammatory response is the body's way to deal with injury or, in the case of allergies and asthma, the intrusion of perceived enemies. When triggered by PAF, other white blood cells and chemicals, called "mediators," rush to the site of the intrusion to quell the disturbance. The best-known mediator is histamine. Histamine causes the most familiar allergic reactions: Released in the nose, eyes, and sinuses, histamine stimulates sneezing, runny nose, and itchy eyes; released in the lungs, it causes symptoms of asthma such as narrowing and swelling of the lining of the airways and the secretion of mucus; in the skin, rashes and hives; and in the digestive system, cramping and diarrhea. It does so by making blood vessels swell and leak fluid into nearby tissues, causing irritation and, often, muscle spasms.

As you'll see, the medications used to treat allergies and asthma—including ginkgo biloba extract—work to limit the inflammatory response by interfering either with the action of PAF or the release of histamine.

UNDERSTANDING ALLERGIES AND ASTHMA

Although scientists know more about the immune system and how it works than ever before, they still do not understand why and how someone develops allergies. Why does it happen that an immune system gets out of whack, hypervigilant and hypersensitive to benign substances? Unfortunately, no one knows the answer to that question. But some of the theories about the causes of allergies, and some of the reasons why allergies seem so much more common today, include the following:

- *Genetics.* It appears that some of us inherit from our parents a susceptibility to the development of allergies. That is not to say that we inherit an allergy to any specific substance. Rather, it seems as if we might inherit some kind of immune system defect or weakness that leaves us more vulnerable to allergies.

- *Overexposure to toxins.* Many scientists believe that the large amount of pollutants to which we are exposed day after day, year after year—in the air we breathe, the food we eat, the water we drink, even the clothes we wear—so disrupts our immune systems that they become hypersensitive and hyperactive, unable to differentiate between harmful and benign substances.

- *Overstimulation by medicines.* The overuse of certain medications, especially antibiotics, may also contribute to the development of allergies. Antibiotics have wide-ranging effects on the body—not all of them positive and many of them leading to or exacerbating allergies. It appears that antibiotics disrupt the internal balance of the body by destroying not only harmful bacteria but "friendly" bacteria as well. Many scientists believe that antibiotic use leads directly to the development of food intolerances and allergies in later life.

- *Emotional stress.* Although a certain amount of stress is a normal part of life, prolonged stress can lead to a depletion and disruption of the immune system. This leaves the body more vulnerable to any number of illnesses and conditions, including an increased susceptibility to allergies.

- *Nutrients.* Many nutrients are involved in the immune response, and imbalances or deficiencies of these nutrients can lead to a malfunction of the immune system, resulting in allergies. Zinc, magnesium, B vitamins, bioflavonoids, and essential fatty acids all can help protect against allergy.

Here, There, Everywhere

There are as many types of allergic reactions as there are allergens and people with allergies. In general, however, allergies are broken down into the following categories:

- *Skin allergies* (including contact dermatitis, atopic dermatitis, and hives). Most people are susceptible to skin allergies or reaction at some point during their lives. Poison ivy and poison oak are the most common culprits, causing itchy, blistering rashes, but almost any substance can cause an allergic reaction in the skin.
- *Respiratory allergies* (including hay fever/allergic rhinitis, allergies to dust, dander, mold, and asthma). Allergies of the respiratory tract most often produce symptoms similar to those of a cold, including congested nasal passages, runny nose, coughing, wheezing, and sneezing. For some people, these symptoms appear only during pollen season. For others, symptoms occur in the winter, when homes and offices are closed to ventilation, causing irritants like dust, molds, mites, and other common airborne allergens to accumulate. Still others experience symptoms whenever they come into contact with furry animals. Although most respiratory allergies—including asthma—represent

responses of the immune system to airborne allergens, allergies to food and chemicals can trigger symptoms as well.

- *Food allergies.* Many people find that certain foods, or combinations of foods, cause their immune system to overreact, leaving them feeling ill and uncomfortable. Symptoms can occur throughout the body and range from a mild stomachache to sudden death. If the reaction occurs when the food moves into the stomach and intestines, nausea, vomiting, bowel crams, or diarrhea may result. The reaction can occur in the respiratory system, causing asthma attacks and breathing problems. Skin symptoms, including hives, itching, and swelling, may also result, as may headaches, irritability, and mood swings.

  Any kind of food—fruits and vegetables, meats and fish, nuts, grains, sugar, caffeine, alcohol, dairy products, and additives and preservatives—can cause an allergic reaction by triggering an immune response or by more subtly undermining the immune system's ability to function properly. However, the most common foods that seem to cause allergic reactions are wheat, dairy, yeast, preservatives, caffeine, corn, and soy.

- *Drug allergies.* Penicillin, Novocain, and streptomycin are among the drugs that may trigger allergic responses, but any drug can cause an immune system overreaction. Symptoms run the gamut from rashes to severe respiratory distress.

- *Chemical inhalant allergies* (i.e., allergies to industrial chemicals, pesticides, synthetics, and air pollution). Paraphenylenediamine, a chemical used in hair and fur dye, leather, rubber, and printing; nickel compounds; rubber compounds; ethylenediamine, a preservative in creams and eye solutions; dichromates used in textile ink, paints and leather; and some chemicals used in antiperspirants and cosmetics are common triggers of allergies (especially skin allergies). Again, the sheer number and diversity of substances we ingest or inhale during the average day is overwhelming—which is why it may be difficult to pinpoint the allergen triggering your symptoms.

The Special Case for Asthma

As discussed earlier, asthma is often considered a type of allergy or, to be more precise, a disease process related to allergy. In some cases, however, the cause of asthma and its triggers remain unknown. No matter the cause, asthma can be a very serious condition: Throughout the 1990s, the occurrence of asthma and deaths due to asthma increased significantly worldwide, probably owing to increased environmental pollution, among other factors. In the United States alone, the incidence of asthma and deaths due to asthma rose 60 percent. Annually, about 500,000 asthma-related hospitalizations occur and about 5,000 people die.

People with asthma have inflamed airways that tend to overreact to any substance that might normally only slightly constrict the bronchial tubes, such as cold air or irritants like cigarette smoke or perfume. Any allergen that enters the respiratory system can also cause this overreaction by the bronchial tubes, thanks in large part to the triggering effect of PAF.

During an asthma attack, the airway linings swell and fill with clogging mucus. The muscles around the bronchial tubes may also constrict, causing severe breathing difficulties and wheezing, a condition known as bronchospasm. If immediate treatment is not applied, death may result.

TREATING ALLERGIES AND ASTHMA

If you have allergies or suffer with asthma, you already know the goal of treatment for these conditions: to alleviate the symptoms and/or to prevent attacks from occurring in the first place. Clearly, the most efficient way of treating allergies is to avoid the triggers altogether. If you know you're allergic to cats, for instance, have your feline-owning companions to your house for dinner rather than risk an attack by visiting them.

Unfortunately, avoiding allergens is almost never easy, and is sometimes downright impossible, which is why over-the-counter and prescription medications for allergies and asthma represent a million-dollar industry—and why a natural remedy like ginkgo biloba is so appealing.

Generally speaking, medications—natural or manmade—for allergies and asthma are designed to reduce the action of histamine (the chemical mediator responsible for most allergy symptoms) and, in the case of asthma, to keep the bronchial tubes as open and clear as possible. Other treatment options include improving your diet, reducing stress, getting regular exercise, and taking supplements of magnesium and vitamin C.

Ginkgo Biloba—The Natural Way

The use of ginkgo biloba extract for the treatment and prevention of allergies and asthma is just starting to gain ground here in the United States. As discussed earlier, GBE helps prevent the overproduction of PAF in the body, thereby reducing both the inflammation (redness, itchiness, heat, and rashes) and the bronchial spasms related to respiratory allergies and asthma.

Several recent studies confirm GBE's positive effects. For a 1990 study published in the *Journal of the American Academy of Dermatology*, scientists first injected 12 patients with PAF and then observed an immediate skin reaction—a hiveslike rash and wheals (raised and itchy patch of skin)—typical of an allergic response. They then treated the patients with 120 mg/day of GBE for several days before repeating the test. The results were remarkable: The hives-and-wheals response was far less pronounced and, in some cases, was completely eliminated.

The findings from one of the most impressive studies of GBE and asthma were published in a 1987 issue of the journal *Prostaglandins*. Here, one group of patients diagnosed with bronchial asthma received 120 mg/day of GBE for three days, while another group received a placebo. The volunteers were then challenged with a spray of house dust mites or pollen allergen. The researchers found that GBE significantly inhibited early bronchoconstriction and showed a tendency to reduce bronchial hyperactivity for up to six hours after exposure to the allergen.

Just as important, GBE produced virtually no side effects, which, as you'll see next, represents a significant benefit over conventional medications. However, it's important to note here, as elsewhere, that GBE is an herbal remedy, which means it exerts its effects on the body slowly, over a period of several days or even weeks. If you currently suffer from allergies and asthma and are taking any medication for your condition, make sure you discuss with your doctor either slowly replacing or supplementing your current medications with GBE.

Conventional Medications

If you've been diagnosed with asthma or allergies, no doubt you're already taking one or more of the following prescription or over-the-counter medications to alleviate your symptoms. Although there appears to be no harm in using these drugs occasionally on a short-term basis, each has its own side effect that can be debilitating and, over the long term, even detrimental to your general health.

- *Antihistamines and decongestants.* The first line of treatment for allergies and asthma usually involves antihistamines, which reduce the action of histamine in the body, and decongestants, which reduce the swelling and stuffiness of the nasal passages. Both of these medications may have unpleasant side effects. Antihistamines frequently cause drowsiness and dizziness, while decongestants often result in nervousness and nausea. If taken over a long period of time, decongestants may have a rebound effect, increasing symptoms rather than decreasing them. People with high blood pressure and vascular disease should avoid decongestants, which are used to relieve the stuffiness associated with allergies, since they tend to constrict blood vessels.
- *Corticosteroids.* These powerful anti-inflammatory drugs come in various forms—injection, capsule, nasal spray, and cream. Available mostly by prescription, they can be useful in treating allergy symptoms but have serious side effects. Muscle weakness, thinning of the skin, high blood pres-

sure, and weight gain are just a few of the common side effects of long-term corticosteroid use.

- *Cromolyn sodium.* A noncorticosteroid drug prescribed mostly for respiratory allergies and asthma, this drug is available in oral form, as a nasal spray, as eyedrops, and in an inhaler. Doctors often prescribe it in advance of the allergy season, because patients must apply it for several weeks before its benefits become apparent—as you'll need to do if you decide to use ginkgo for your allergies. Cromolyn works by preventing IgE from leaving the mast cells where they reside, and therefore lessening the allergic response.

- *Immunotherapy.* This treatment attempts to desensitize the immune system. Your doctor will give you a series of injections containing the allergen over a period of several months. In theory, you will become less allergic to the offending substance as time goes on and your body adjusts to it. However, the process is a long and expensive one, and one that fails to solve the problem in more than 30 percent of cases.

Other Herbal Remedies to Try

As discussed earlier, herbal medicines generally work in much the same way as conventional pharmaceuticals do: They contain substances that work to alter the body's chemistry in order to return it to its natural state of health. Unlike purified drugs, however, plants and other organic materials tend to be less potentially toxic to the body and thus cause fewer side effects.

If you decide to take ginkgo biloba or other herbs to treat your allergies or asthma symptoms, it's important for you to seek guidance from an herbalist or other experienced professional practitioner of alternative medicine. He or she will attempt to prescribe the right combination of herbs and other therapies for your particular symptoms and constitution. In the meantime, here are a few suggestions:

- *Goldenseal.* Also known as yellow root, goldenseal helps to dry up and soothe mucous membranes throughout the body, which makes it especially useful in alleviating congestion in both the respiratory and digestive tracts. It is sold as capsules (taken 2 to 5 times daily), as a tincture (½ to 1 teaspoon a day), or in powdered form for consumption as a tea.
- *Cayenne.* Also known as hot red pepper, cayenne is one of the most useful herbal remedies for allergies and asthma. Its active ingredient, capsaicin, is a strong anti-inflammatory, helping to soothe burning nasal passages, bronchial tubes, and lungs. Cayenne is also a good digestive tonic and benefits the heart and circulation. It is rich in vitamin C and other antioxidants. As a powder, cayenne can be used in food or drunk as a tea. You can also derive benefits by eating hot spicy foods made with cayenne pepper, as you may have already experienced.
- *Echinacea.* Also known as purple cornflower, this plant is a traditional Native American remedy known to have extraordinary immune system–boosting qualities. Many clinical and laboratory studies document the ability of echinacea to strengthen body tissue and protect against invasive allergens. You can use echinacea in many forms: capsule (1 capsule up to 3 times a day), tincture (1 teaspoon up to 3 times a day), and extract (mix 15

to 30 drops in water or juice and take up to 4 times a day).

Eat for a Healthy Immune System

Creating a healthy diet isn't important only for those with specific food sensitivities but for everyone who suffers from allergies. Here are a few tips:

- *Maintain a healthy weight.* Many people with food allergies tend to be underweight (because they attempt to eliminate too many foods in order to alleviate their symptoms) or overweight (because they tend to overindulge in food to which they are unknowingly allergic). Drugs used to treat chronic asthma and allergies may also cause weight gain.
- *Eat foods that leave you feeling healthy and well.* In addition to avoiding foods to which you are allergic, it's important to recognize that you may be sensitive in more subtle ways to other kinds—or amounts—of food. Pay attention to how you feel after your meals. If you're often groggy and uncomfortable, you may be eating too much, failing to eat a balanced diet, or consuming food that doesn't agree with your particular body makeup. Nutritious food, prepared well and eaten in a relaxed atmosphere, should nourish your body and soul. The best way to identify a food that is causing a reaction is to eliminate a suspected food for three weeks, then add it back into the diet. If the elimination of the food alleviated the problem, and returning it brought back symptoms, you've found the culprit.
- *Be alert to the potential dangers of sugar and yeast.* If you suffer from allergies of any kind, pay special

attention to sugar and yeast. Double-blind studies have shown that many people have allergic reactions to refined cane sugar. Furthermore, sugar and other simple carbohydrates tend to feed another substance in the body that can wreak havoc on our immune system: yeast. Yeast (particularly the species known as *Candida albicans*) is a substance that lives in our bodies naturally, primarily in the mouth, esophagus, intestines, vagina, and skin. As long as our immune system keeps it in balance, *Candida* levels stay in check. However, should the immune system become weak for any reason, the yeast can multiply, forming colonies that further challenge the immune system. New research shows that chronic yeast infection may lead someone to develop severe allergies to inhalants (like pollen and ragweed), foods of all kinds, medications, and chemicals. In fact, the person who is sensitive to a wide variety of substances is more likely to have an allergy to yeast, or have a chronic yeast infection, than is someone sensitive to just one or two allergens.

In addition to these general dietary recommendations, you may also want to consider the benefit of increasing the amount of certain vitamins and minerals in your diet. Of particular interest to those who suffer with allergies and asthma are the following:

- *Zinc.* Studies in laboratory animals and in humans have shown that deficiencies in this trace mineral depress the immune system, leaving the body vulnerable to both allergies and infections. Zinc plays an important role in the production of IgA, the gastrointestinal antibody found in saliva and in the digestive tract. When IgA binds to an allergen, it keeps it from being absorbed into the bloodstream and thus from causing an allergic reaction. You can get more zinc in your diet by either taking supplements or by boosting your intake of zinc-rich foods like meat, liver, eggs, and seafood.

- *Vitamin A.* Vitamin A also acts to increase the body's production of IgA, thus helping to reduce the immune system reactions to food and other allergens. Liver, eggs, carrots, tomatoes, and fish are particularly rich sources of vitamin A.

- *Flavonoids.* Another reason ginkgo biloba is so terrific at treating allergies is that it is filled with antioxidants known as flavonoids, which serve to modify the human body's reaction to allergens and inhibit the inflammatory response. The most important types of flavonoids for people with allergies are those found in blueberries, blackberries, cherries, and grapes. Like those found in ginkgo, these flavonoids help to decrease the leakiness and fragility of small blood vessels, as well as protect against free-radical damage.

Maintaining a healthy diet is one part of creating an allergy-free—or at least allergy-reduced—lifestyle. Two other components are related: reducing your stress levels and exercising.

Reduce Stress and Exercise!

Believe it or not, there exists a direct connection between emotional well-being and susceptibility to allergies. This connection involves stress: the body's response to any stimulus that interferes with its normal functioning. Any exciting external circumstance can be a stress-provoking event, from a joyful event like the birth of a child to a personal crisis like the loss of a job. And any internal adjustments your body must make in an effort to keep its chemistry and biology in good working order involve a certain amount of stress. If you fail to eat a proper diet, for instance, you challenge your body to keep itself up and running despite a lack of nutrients.

As discussed in Chapter 4, the most well known reaction to stress is the "fight-or-flight response." When faced with a difficult or threatening challenge, the body releases certain chemicals that cause the respiration, blood pressure, and heart rates to rise, muscles to tense, and senses to heighten. One challenge that can cause this response is an allergy or asthma attack. No doubt you become more anxious when you realize that your skin is breaking out, your eyes are watering, or your bronchial tubes are swelling in reaction to an allergen. Unfortunately, this set of responses does nothing to help you avoid the attack. In fact, it may work to make the attack worse by heightening the symptoms—increasing respiration, for instance, or triggering a rash. In addition, the longer your body remains under stress, the less healthy your immune system will be, which leaves you more vulnerable to future allergy attacks or even to developing new sensitivities.

In order to break the cycle of stress→allergy/asthma attack→more stress→more attacks, you should first try to find a way to reduce the amount of tension and anxiety you feel on a day-to-day basis. We discuss these methods—which include meditation, biofeedback, and progressive relaxation—in Chapter 8. Please see pages 175–182 for some tips on how to reduce your stress levels.

In addition, we must emphasize here the importance

of regular exercise to your general health. Although exercise won't clear your lungs or realign your immune system, without regular exercise, your body simply can't function in balance and health. In addition to reducing your risk of developing heart disease stroke, high blood pressure, some kinds of cancer, and a myriad of other diseases, exercise can dramatically improve the quality of your life. Exercising on a regular basis will help you look better and increase your feelings of self-esteem. It will help you release physical and emotional tension and anxiety, as well as build up your stamina and strength. If nothing else, regular exercise will help you feel more empowered and less like a helpless victim to allergy and asthma attacks.

In addition, exercise has been shown to stabilize the production of stress hormones and thus help to control the allergic response. Other body chemicals stimulated by exercise are endorphins and enkephalins, which have mood-elevating effects, helping to reduce stress, irritability, and pain.

Perhaps you've shied away from physical activity because you're afraid that stressing your body in this way may increase your risk of having an allergy attack. If you have asthma and respiratory symptoms of allergies, exercising—particularly outside—may well have triggered an allergy attack in the past. If so, it is important that you talk to your doctor about finding safe, healthful ways to get your blood pumping and your muscles working so that you can stay well throughout your life. In the end, moderate exercise will only serve to make you feel stronger and in more control of your allergies and their symptoms. For more tips about making exercise a regular part of your life, see Chapter 8.

Of course, exercise benefits the cardiovascular system most. It opens up the blood vessels, increasing circulation throughout the body. This effect is important not only in the prevention of heart disease but, as you'll see, in very special aspects of the health of men and women.

Find Out More About . . .

. . . Ginkgo Biloba and Allergies

Q. Will a single dose of ginkgo help an asthma or allergy attack, or do I need to take it for a longer period of time for it to have an effect?

A. Because allergies develop over a period of time, long-term use of ginkgo is the most effective way to prevent an allergic reaction, because excessive PAF production will be continually blocked and will become relevant whenever you are exposed to an allergen. If ginkgo biloba is already working on your system before you are exposed to a potential allergen, the response of PAF tends to be far less intensive.

At the same time, then it's important to remember that GBE is NOT a particularly good way to reduce allergy or asthma symptoms once a full-fledged attack begins. That's where conventional medications like antihistamines and decongestants come in handy, as do other herbs (especially cayenne).

Q. If I take ginkgo biloba supplements regularly, will my allergies or asthma be cured?

A. Almost certainly not. No cure for allergies or asthma currently exists. Taking GBE on a regular basis, however, will certainly help alleviate your symptoms and help protect lung and other tissue from becoming damaged by excess and chronic inflammation.

. . . Allergies

Q. Might I suddenly develop an allergy to something that never bothered me before?

A. Yes. In fact, technically, all allergies develop this way. You may exist for years before ever coming into frequent contact with, say, strawberries, but once you start eating them regularly, you may develop a severe reaction. Or you may live your entire life with a dog, but "suddenly" become allergic when your body has developed enough IgE antibodies to begin producing PAF and setting off the chain of events that lead to unpleasant symptoms of inflammation.

Q. My doctor thinks I suffer from "leaky gut" syndrome. What is this condition, and what does it have to do with my allergies?

A. Leaky gut syndrome is a condition in which your digestive tract is more permeable than it should be. In other words, it allows partially digested food particles to pass through the digestive tract and, once in the bloodstream, to trigger an immune system reaction. This may cause an allergic response to that particular substance or cause the immune system to become overstimulated in general, leaving the body more vulnerable to allergies of all kinds. Because ginkgo biloba also helps reduce the permeability of blood vessels, it may be an especially helpful treatment for your condition. Mention it to your doctor or nutritionist.

Q. My allergies are just horrible during the spring and fall. What can I do to avoid having such a bad time of it?

A. In addition to taking GBE, you can also learn to better avoid the triggers of your attacks. The American Lung Association makes the following recommendations:

• *Monitor air quality.* Listen to media reports about your local pollen count. Allergy symptoms most often develop when pollen counts are moderate to high, but can continue even when the count lowers. Rainy, cloudy, or windless days usually have lower pollen counts, but mold spores may be higher soon after rainfall. Taking note of which allergens are at the highest levels when you are troubled by allergies may help you narrow down your triggers, and plan your activities for better times.

• *Avoid early-morning activity.* Pollen levels are highest before 10 A.M., so try not to be outdoors then. While indoors, close windows and use air-conditioning to filter and dry the air.

• *Dry your clothes and sheets indoors.* Do not hang linens or clothing outside to dry. Pollen and molds collect on these materials and can trigger allergies later.

• *Limit alcohol intake.* Alcohol stimulates mucus production and dilates blood vessels, worsening runny nose and nasal congestion.

• *Stop smoking.* If for no other reason than to alleviate your allergy symptoms, put out your last cigarette. Smoking irritates the eyes and respiratory system, making symptoms worse.

Q. I've heard of the herb "ma huang" as a treatment for asthma. Is it safe to use?

A. Ma huang, or ephedra, is a Chinese herb that dilates the breathing passages and shrinks blood vessels. In fact, the decongestant medications ephedrine and pseudo-ephedrine, found in many over-the-counter remedies, work in similar ways. Because ma huang shrinks blood vessels, however, it can be risky to take, especially in people who also have high blood pressure and heart disease. In general, then, it should be used only under the guidance of a quali-fied health practitioner.

Q. My son has what the doctor calls "exercise-induced asthma. Does this mean he shouldn't play sports?

A. Exercise is one of the most common triggers of asthma in children and young adults. In fact, more than 80 percent of people with asthma wheeze or cough when they exercise or experience some degree of tightness in the chest. If you're trying to solve your son's problem with a natural medicine like ginkgo biloba, which may take longer to work than mainstream solutions, your son may need to cut down on activities—at least until his most severe symp-toms are alleviated. You may also want to consider having him use conventional medications just on those days he participates in strenuous physical activity. For many chil-dren, cromolyn sodium taken a half hour before exercise allows them to play a game of soccer, football, or other sport without becoming ill. Talk to your doctor about it.

CHAPTER 6

Ginkgo for Women,
Ginkgo for Men

Circulation. It's a concept we're most used to thinking about in connection with our hearts and brains, but rarely with our sex lives or hormonal cycles. In fact, however, how well your body delivers its supply of blood and other nutrients, and picks up waste products and excess fluid, has a definite impact on your health. For a woman, a lack of proper circulation may exacerbate premenstrual syndrome—a group of debilitating symptoms related to her menstrual cycle. For men, poor circulation can lead to impotence—the inability to achieve and sustain an erection. Clearly, each problem has a very different set of causes, effects, and treatments. What's remarkable is that ginkgo biloba extract in a standard dose of about 120 mg/day can help alleviate both conditions. Let's take them one by one, starting with women first.

PREMENSTRUAL SYNDROME

In *The Sickness of Virgins,* Hippocrates ascribed a variety of symptoms, including delusions, mania, and thoughts of suicide, to "retained menstrual blood"— perhaps the first reference to a medical constellation of symptoms we now know as premenstrual syndrome, or PMS. According to the Premenstrual Institute, up to 40 percent of women of childbearing age suffer from some degree of premenstrual syndrome. Sometimes PMS begins with the first menstruation, but sometimes it doesn't appear until after a woman has given birth for the first time, experienced some sort of gynecological surgery, or is experiencing a period of major stress. PMS may be hereditary and may become worse with age as hormonal fluctuations become more marked.

Among the symptoms involved in this syndrome are the following:

- *Physical symptoms:* bloating, swollen/painful breasts, swollen hands and feet, weight gain, food cravings, headaches, skin problems, dizziness.
- *Emotional problems:* short temper, aggression, anger, anxiety/panic, confusion, depression, lack of concentration

The one consistent complaint among women suffering from PMS is the cyclical nature of symptoms. PMS symptoms appear during the week before a woman's period (or when a woman ovulates), begin to subside with the onset of menstruation, and are absent during the week following menstruation. (If you're unsure if your symptoms are related to your monthly cycle, start keeping a diary. Track both your symptoms and your periods to see if a pattern develops.)

Premenstrual syndrome, or PMS, is a difficult condition to diagnose because of the wide variety of symptoms and the complicated systems involved. Indeed, the regulation of the menstrual cycle involves complex interactions among neurotransmitters (the brain's chemical messengers) and hormones. These interactions prompt a number of physical changes affecting almost every organ system in the body and, for many women, cause uncomfortable symptoms in the two weeks before their periods begin. Before we discuss what might be going wrong, let's examine what happens during a normal cycle.

Understanding the Cycle

A female child is born with ovaries that are completely stocked with all the eggs she'll ever have—about one million. During her fertile life, a woman will release just 300 to 400 eggs, one each month for about 35 to 40 years. The rest simply atrophy. Each egg, which is little more than a dot of fluid packed with genetic information, is encapsulated in a tiny sac called a follicle and lodged within ovarian tissue. Every month, the body prepares one egg (and occasionally two or more) for fertilization and the uterus for a potential pregnancy. This preparation is known as the menstrual cycle.

Although by definition a cycle has no beginning or end, for description purposes let's assign the starting position of the menstrual cycle to the hypothalamus, an endocrine gland in the brain. At the beginning of the cycle the hypothalamus sends a message in the form of a hormone called gonadotropin-releasing hormone (GnRH) to the pituitary gland. The pituitary, which is located just below the hypothalamus, then relays its own message to the ovaries by another hormone called the follicle-stimulating hormone (FSH).

Stimulation from FSH causes one of the follicles in one of the ovaries to grow and the ovum within it to mature. At the same time, a thick layer of cells covers the follicle and ovum: These cells secrete the hormone estradiol, a type of estrogen. The estrogen is released into the bloodstream and acts on the lining of the uterus, called the endometrium, causing it to grow and thicken in preparation for the arrival of a fertilized egg. This occurs during the first part of the cycle, called the estrogen phase, which takes about 14 days.

At this time, the hypothalamus, stimulated by the elevated levels of estrogen in the bloodstream, signals the pituitary to secrete a second hormone, known as luteinizing hormone (LH). The surge of LH causes the developing follicle to enlarge and rupture. In the event known as ovulation, the mature ovum is then expelled into the fallopian tubes and makes its way up into the uterus, a journey that takes about six days. While it is in transit, sperm can fertilize the egg if it is present.

In the meantime, the remnant follicle in the ovary is transformed into a working endocrine gland called the corpeus luteum. The corpus luteum produces both estrogen and large quantities of progesterone, the female hormone dominant in the second half of the cycle, known as the luteal phase. Under the impact of progesterone, the cells in the uterine lining grow and mature further. By the end of the menstrual cycle, the endometrium has doubled in thickness, and large amounts of nutrients meant to nourish a fetus have been stored there.

If sperm fertilizes the egg, the fertilized egg implants itself into the lining of the endometrium and a special hormone, called chorionic gonadotropin, is secreted to stimulate the continued production of estrogen and progesterone. In fact, the egg itself becomes its very own hormone-producing factory. Without fertilization and continued hormone secretion, on the other hand, the corpus luteum begins to shrink and levels of estrogen and progesterone drop. When the hormonal level is at its lowest, the uterus sheds its lining and the menstrual period begins. By the fourth or fifth day of the period, hormone levels have dropped enough to signal the hypothalamus to resume the process. Unless interrupted by pregnancy, surgical removal of the ovaries, or a hormonal imbalance caused by illness or stress, this remarkable cycle continues throughout a woman's fertile life.

What Goes Wrong

Sounds organized and straightforward, doesn't it? Unfortunately, and for reasons scientists still do not fully understand, some women's bodies react badly to these hormonal fluctuations. One theory is that the pituitary gland, which regulates hormone release throughout the body, may be sending out the wrong messages, which can lead to a hormone imbalance in certain women.

Some researchers, including Susan Lark, M.D., in her book *PMS Self-Help Book,* divide women with PMS into several subgroups depending on their particular symptoms and their suggested triggers, though many women fall into more than one category. Let's take a look:

- *PMS-A.* These women tend to experience high levels of anxiety, irritability, and mood swings, which may be related to higher levels of estrogen and lower levels of progesterone.

- *PMS-C.* This subgroup of women experience increased appetite and crave carbohydrates, perhaps because they have lower levels of serotonin. This group tend to suffer from headaches and dizziness as well.
- *PMS-D.* Women in this category tend to be depressed and forgetful during their premenstrual phase, which is perhaps related to higher levels of progesterone and lower levels of estrogen than usual.
- *PMS-H.* Fluid retention, weight gain, swollen extremities, breast tenderness, and abdominal bloating are the symptoms suffered by women in this subgroup. And it is these women who may benefit the most from taking ginkgo biloba.

TREATING PMS

Like many conditions whose causes aren't completely understood, PMS can be treated with varying degrees of success. Some women will experience symptom relief by taking anti-inflammatory drugs such as ibuprofen. getting more sleep, and avoiding certain possible dietary triggers such as sugar, salt, caffeine, and alcohol. For others, going on birth control pills or taking antidepressants may be helpful. Let's take a look at some of these alternatives.

The Ginkgo Solution

Bloating, breast tenderness, swelling of the hands and feet, muscle aches and pains . . . These are among the symptoms of PMS directly related to fluid retention and vascular congestion experienced by women in the

PMS-H category. Researchers believe that menstrual-related fluid retention and swelling may be caused by an increase in capillary permeability and vascular congestion, triggered by hormonal changes.

Since GBE has been shown to normalize excessive capillary permeability, relieve vascular congestion, and restore circulation to all tissues, it isn't surprising that taking it could alleviate PMS. The body will keep blood and lymph flowing more efficiently, eliminating the buildup of fluid in tissues. In one study of 10 women experiencing menstrual-related swelling in which the women were all given GBE, three women experienced the complete disappearance of edema, while six others showed significant improvement. All 10 women experienced a correction of their abnormal capillary permeability.

A more rigorous double-blind study involved 165 women between 18 and 45 years of age who had experienced symptoms of edema for at least three menstrual cycles. They were given either 80 milligrams of GBE twice daily or a placebo from the sixteenth day of one menstrual cycle to the fifth day of the text. After a complete evaluation of symptoms, researchers determined that those patients receiving GBE extract experienced significantly more symptom relief, especially relief of breast-related symptoms such as pain and swelling.

The same study also noted improvements in the neuropsychological conditions of those taking GBE over those taking the placebo. Ginkgo has been shown to have a positive effect on headaches, dizziness, and depression, so again, it isn't surprising that it should help to relieve these symptoms when they are associated with PMS.

Conventional Medication

Since no one is quite certain what causes PMS, it should come as no surprise that your regular doctor can offer no simple solution to ease your discomfort. Besides recommending that you take ibuprofen, an anti-inflammatory known to help the cramping and discomfort associated with PMS, your doctor will probably suggest some of the lifestyle changes we recommend next—mainly improving your diet by avoiding certain substances (salt, caffeine, sugar, and fat) while increasing your intake of specific vitamins and minerals (particularly vitamin B complex, calcium, and beta-carotene). Vitamin E can also be helpful.

If your case of PMS is particularly severe, your doctor may prescribe oral contraceptives, which help regulate and moderate the amount of hormones throughout the cycle. If you suffer from debilitating mood swings—a frequent symptom—you may benefit from one of the selective serotonin-reuptake inhibitors (SSRIs) often used to treat depression, including Prozac, Paxil, and Zoloft, among others.

A Healthy Diet

A very enlightening study, published in a 1982 issue of the *Journal of Applied Nutrition,* examined the dietary patterns of 39 women with PMS compared with 14 women who did not suffer from the symptoms. The results: Those with PMS all consumed more refined sugar, refined carbohydrates, and dairy products than those without the problem. Healthy women consumed considerably more B vitamins, iron, zinc, manganese, and niacin—up to 45 times more, in fact.

In addition to eating a healthy, balanced diet such as

the one described in Chapter 8, here are some tips that may help alleviate your symptoms:

- *Learn to graze.* Many experts suggest sticking to smaller, more frequent meals while experiencing PMS. Don't eat more—just divide up the food you would normally eat into six meals instead of three.
- *Go for the pure and simple.* Fresh fruits and vegetables, whole grains, and proteins low in fat are sensible choices. Avoid processed foods and foods high in saturated fats.
- *Go for the carbs.* Eating complex carbohydrates helps to raise serotonin levels, which will boost your mood during this stressful time. Whole-grain cereals, breads, and pastas; rice (preferably brown rice); sweet potatoes; and vegetables are appropriate choices. As tempting as they might sound, avoid simple sugars like those found in cakes and candies.

Exercise

No one is sure why exercise helps PMS symptoms, but it does. Many experts suggest it's the increase in endorphins that accompanies vigorous exercise. These chemicals are natural opiates that provide a sense of well-being while reducing pain. Indeed, one study found that women's endorphin levels dropped during the two weeks before menstruation—just when PMS symptoms occur. Another study connects a drop in endorphin levels with fluid retention and breast tenderness. Finally, regular aerobic exercise may help the body to break down estrogen, which some researchers believe plays a role in PMS.

GINKGO AND IMPOTENCE

Thanks to the recent approval by the FDA of the oral medication Viagra, the word "impotence" has become less taboo. Nevertheless, if you've experienced impotence, you may have been loath to admit it, let alone seek treatment. You aren't alone. Approximately 25 to 30 million American men suffer from impotence, yet according to the Impotence Resource Center, only 5 percent ever seek treatment, an unfortunate fact since almost 95 percent of impotence cases can be successfully treated.

Impotence, also known as erectile dysfunction, is the inability to achieve or maintain an erection during sexual intercourse. It is important to realize that an occasional episode of impotence happens to most men, is perfectly normal, and is no cause for alarm. When it proves to be a pattern or a persistent problem, impotence can be a sign of a medical disorder as well as become a detriment to a man's self-image and sex life. Before we discuss what can go wrong to create this problem, let's take a look at the way an erection normally occurs.

When It Works

A natural erection is the result of a complex process, the center of which is the brain. There, sensations of sexual arousal are first experienced. The brain then sends its arousal signals to the penile nerves. Penile nerves are also stimulated by direct sensory contact, such as manual stroking of the genitalia and by the act of sexual intercourse itself. These nerve impulses go to two "erection chambers" called the corpora cavernosa, causing relaxation of penile tissue and expansion of the arterial blood vessels leading to the penis. Under normal circumstances, blood flow into the erection chambers increases as penile tissue relaxes and penile arteries expand. Veins that normally drain the blood flow are compressed against the inner wall, trapping the blood and making the penis hard and erect.

In a process as complex as penile erection, problems can occur for many reasons. The causes may be psychological or physical or a combination of both. Psychological causes include temporary or chronic stress and anxiety due to financial, relationship, or other external problems. In more than half of all cases, however, the problem is physical. The most frequent physical cause of erectile dysfunction are vascular diseases, which may cause problems involving blood flow into the penis to make it erect or holding blood in the penis to maintain an erection. Simply put, the problem starts when the vascular tissues of the genitalia aren't able to dilate sufficiently to let in enough blood, and/or a sufficient amount of blood fails to reach the penis— even though the brain is sending out the proper signals. Fortunately, treatment is available to help almost everyone with erectile dysfunction. The first step for most men is erasing the negative stereotypes and myths about this common condition.

The Myths About Impotence

Impotence is a normal consequence of aging. Untrue! Most men should be able to enjoy normal sexual relations well into old age, and aging alone should never be considered a reason to accept impotence. However, many diseases, including arteriosclerosis and diabetes, occur at a greater rate as we age.

It's all in your head. In fact, only 15 percent of impotence can be attributed to psychological causes. Usually, it is a secondary condition brought on by physical conditions. As discussed earlier, erectile dysfunction can be the first sign of vascular disease, which could lead to heart attack or stroke—and which is why taking ginkgo can help. It may also be a sign of diabetes. Indeed, diabetes and impotence often go hand in hand. Forty percent of impotence sufferers are diabetic, and 50 percent of diabetic males over the age of fifty experience impotence.

Vascular diseases such as arteriosclerosis, heart disease, and stroke may all result in impotence. One study reported that 39 percent of heart disease patients suffered from impotence, and patients on drugs to treat their heart disease, such as vasodilators and other cardiac drugs, also experienced a high rate of impotence. Another study found that 57 percent of patients undergoing coronary surgery experienced subsequent bouts with impotence.

Spinal cord, brain, pelvic, or groin injuries may damage blood flow to the genitalia, resulting in impotence. More than 200 prescription drugs are known to cause the condition. Even a history of smoking may result in impotence due to the negative effects on the arteries of the penis, which can inhibit blood flow.

Impotence is permanent. As we've said, impotence is a highly treatable condition, which may be addressed in a number of ways, depending on the cause. If your impotence turns out to be psychological in origin, your doctor may prescribe personal or couples counseling for you and/or your partner. In the event it turns out to be physical in origin, treating the underlying disease often resolves the problem. In other cases, medication (both pharmaceutical and herbal) can improve the situation. In particularly stubborn cases, a doctor may recommend surgery and/or the use of a penile implant and other devices, as we'll discuss later in the chapter.

DIAGNOSING IMPOTENCE

If you or your partner suffers erectile dysfunction, it's important to seek help from your doctor. To find the cause, your doctor will take your medical and sexual history. For the medical history, you'll be asked about illnesses such as heart disease, diabetes, depression, and high blood pressure—and any medication you may be taking. Indeed, many medications used to treat those very diseases may themselves trigger impotence.

Included in the sexual history part of the exam are questions dealing with how often you have intercourse, if you wake up with an erection (which indicates the problem may be psychological rather than physical in origin), and whether or not erections are painful for you. Your answers will help the doctor further narrow down the cause.

The next step is the physical exam. Your doctor will pay particular attention to the genitalia and will test nervous and vascular function. He or she may also perform a rectal examination to check the condition of your prostate. Samples of your blood and urine will be sent to a lab for analysis, in order to rule out diabetes and elevated cholesterol levels. If necessary, special tests may also be conducted, such as an ultrasound examination to check the condition of penile arteries. Another kind of special test measures "nocturnal penile tumescence and rigidity," or the number and strength of erections you experience while you're asleep at night. Special gauges are attached to the penis to measure the normal erections that take place during REM sleep (the dreaming portion). If no nocturnal erections occur, then the cause of impotence is likely to be a physical one.

TREATMENT OF IMPOTENCE

Once you've narrowed down the source of the problem, you can start treatment. Fortunately, there are several options for you and your doctor to consider. If psychological problems such as stress, depression, or marital problems are to blame, your doctor will most likely recommend that you seek psychological counseling. If a particular medication is causing your problem, your doctor will work with you to find an alternative that does not affect your ability to achieve or maintain an erection. This option is particularly important if you're taking an antidepressant like Prozac, which frequently has sexual dysfunction as a side effect.

The Ginkgo Solution

Almost every medical condition ginkgo biloba successfully addresses is due, at least in part, to poor circulation, and impotence is certainly no exception. Because GBE successfully enhances circulation and dilates veins and arteries without increasing blood pressure, GBE can often successfully restore healthy circulation to those suffering from impotence.

One study confirming this effect involved 60 patients suffering from impotence due to impaired blood flow who had failed to respond to conventional treatment. All were given 60 mg/day of GBE for 12 to 18 months, and penile blood flow was evaluated monthly via sonography. After just six to eight weeks, some patients showed signs of improved blood flow, and after six months of GBE therapy, fully half the patients in the study had regained erectile function. Twenty percent of those patients who hadn't regained potency now re-acted positively to other medical treatment. In 25 per-cent of the patients who still showed no improvement, sonography showed improved blood flow to the penis, suggesting that they might eventually regain normal function. Only 5 percent of study participants showed no improvement at all.

Although this study wasn't a double-blind study and therefore was considered less rigorous than some (espe-cially since impotence often has a psychological compo-nent), the evidence certainly suggests that GBE can have a dramatic and positive effect on erectile dysfunction. Long-term use of ginkgo biloba in the standard dosage of 120 mg per day, taken in three dosages of 40 mg each, will probably be the most effective treatment of penile blood flow problems.

The Mainstream Approach

In 1998 the FDA approved the first oral treatment for male impotence. Called sildenafil, or Viagra, the tablet is taken one to two hours before sexual activity to achieve an erection satisfactory for intercourse. Viagra works by increasing the amount of time a natural brain chemical (cyclic GMP) is available to achieve or main-tain an erection. Cyclic GMP relaxes specific muscles and allows the blood to flow to the penis. Side effects appear to be mild and relatively rare, but they include stomach upset, nasal congestion, flushing, headaches, and visual disturbances. The other most common treat-ments for impotence caused by an underlying physical (rather than psychological) problem are vacuum therapy, self-injection therapy, and penile implants (either prosthetic or medicinal).

Vacuum therapy is the safest, least expensive, and least invasive treatment. It has the highest success rate—about 75 to 90 percent. Vacuum therapy consists of applying a vacuum device to the penis, which puts it under negative pressure, drawing blood into the area. A band or tension ring is then applied to the base of the penis to maintain the erection, and removed up to 30 minutes later. Some of the problems with vacuum therapy include the necessity of interrupting sexual activity, and in a few cases, discomfort. Because of its benefits, however, it remains a popular option. About 150,000 vacuum devices are prescribed annually.

Self-injection therapy involves injecting medication into the base of the penis. The medications used are vasoactive drugs that relax tissues and encourage blood flow into the area. Erections usually occur within five to 15 minutes and can last for over an hour. Common drug choices include prostaglandin-E1 (PGE1) or drug combinations such as papavarine and phentolamine. The risks of these medications are slight but include the possibility of scarring after long-term use and prolonged erections lasting over four hours (erections lasting too long can damage the penis and medical treatment must be sought). Those who find it difficult to give themselves injections may find this option unpleasant; in addition, these drugs may be used only two to three times per week. Another, newer form of medication is a pellet implanted via an applicator into the urethra. The medication has an effect similar to that of injection, and an erection occurs within five to 10 minutes of insertion of the pellet.

A prosthetic device is a more permanent solution. Because surgery is required to insert the prosthesis, this treatment is the most invasive and usually a last resort, although prosthetic implants have a high satisfaction rate—about 83 percent. Two main types of implants exist: semi-rigid cylinders and inflatable cylinders with a pump implanted in the scrotum. Sexual activity will feel normal and orgasm will be unaffected, but normal function is almost never restored if the device is removed. About 21,000 penile implants are prescribed annually.

Lifestyle Modifications

A good diet and nutritional program is as important to your genitourinary tract as it is to your cardiovascular system. Generally speaking, in fact, you should follow the same healthy diet prescription recommended in Chapters 4 and 8, which are designed to keep your blood vessels clear and functioning well, your blood pressure normal, and your immune system alert and ready to fight against harmful viruses and bacteria.

FIND OUT MORE ABOUT . . .

. . . Premenstrual Syndrome

Q. You wrote that women with PMS frequently have lower than normal levels of serotonin. Isn't that the substance related to depression?

A. Yes, and there appears to be a direct connection between hormones produced by the ovaries and serotonin, the neurotransmitter most related to depression. In women who suffer from PMS, serotonin levels drop precipitously during the week before menstruation.

This serotonin depletion helps explain two common symptoms of PMS: mood swings and cravings for carbohydrates (substances that naturally boost serotonin levels in the brain). In fact, studies show that women with PMS eat an average of 500 extra carbohydrate calories per day in the week before their periods.

. . . Impotence

Q. I'm so embarrassed to admit I've been experiencing impotence that I'd almost rather live with it than tell anyone. What's the harm?

A. First of all, it would be a shame if embarrassment were the sole reason for denying yourself a satisfying sex life. As discussed, impotence is far more common than you might think, and thus doctors have attained a great deal of experience in dealing with the problem in a sensitive and straightforward manner. Second, because impotence could signal a number of physical health problems—it may even be the very first sign of impending heart disease, stroke, or diabetes—your life could depend on getting an accurate diagnosis. By receiving prompt treatment, you can avoid serious disability and even death. If a psychological problem lies at the root of your difficulties, there's a good chance that you're experiencing difficulties in other areas of your life—your job, your marriage, your self-esteem. Undergoing some short-term psychotherapy can make a marked difference. We strongly urge that you put aside your feelings of embarrassment and talk to your doctor as soon as possible.

Q. My partner takes my impotence personally. I've told her it has nothing to do with her, but she doesn't believe me. What should I do?

A. For anyone involved in a sexual relationship, impotence is a couples problem. Women want and need sex, too, and when something goes wrong in the sexual arena, your partner will naturally wonder if it might have something to do with her.

And maybe it does. If you are experiencing marital problems, your body may not comply with your mind's requests, knowing that something is amiss. More than likely, however, you have a medical or psychiatric problem that requires treatment, and with that treatment, your potency problems will be resolved.

If you feel comfortable, ask your wife to accompany you to the doctor to discuss the cause and effect of impotence. If the doctor finds evidence that the cause is psychological, consider attending counseling sessions together. You may find you have been blaming her for your impotence, even if she wasn't the initial cause. If you are in a serious relationship, any problem of yours is a problem of hers, too. Because for men sexual prowess and self-esteem are so closely linked, one or two temporary bouts with impotence can initiate a downward spiral of a man's self-esteem, perpetuating impotence that needn't continue. In other words, you're afraid you won't be able to perform, so your body obliges your fears. Allowing your partner to help you explore your sexual or stress issues will help both of you. Working together in this manner can enrich your relationship and, eventually, improve your sex life.

CHAPTER 7

Keeping the Senses Alive

- Bob had been suffering from tinnitus—a disturbing and unexplainable ringing in his years—for several years. His doctor couldn't offer any relief, and the condition seemed to be getting worse. After reading about ginkgo biloba extract, Bob went to an herbalist recommended to him by a friend. The herbalist suggested that he take 120 mg per day of GBE. Three months later, Bob experiences far fewer episodes of tinnitus, and they tend to be far milder than those he had earlier.
- Sixty-eight-year-old Conseula found out from her doctor that she's in the very early stages of diabetic retinopathy, an eye disease threatening her vision. Related to her diabetes mellitus, this condition can be progressive, and represents another major cause of blindness. After working out a new treatment plan to better her control over her blood sugar, Consuela decided to take ginkgo biloba extract to help protect her vision. Nearly a year later, her doctor has told her that the disease has not progressed

and she won't need surgery in the foreseeable future.

- Tom, 76, also started taking ginkgo biloba when he heard about its vision-saving qualities. He recently watched as his wife's vision declined due to age-related macular degeneration, a progressive eye disease that represents the most common cause of visual loss among the elderly in the United States. Since his vision was not impaired when he started taking ginkgo, he hasn't noticed a change in that area. He does report feeling a renewed sense of energy and a strengthened ability to concentrate and focus.

- Janna is 38 years old and has experienced chronic dizziness for more than three years. Her doctor thinks she may have a disorder of the inner ear, but can't track down the source of the problem. In the meantime, she's decided to take ginkgo biloba after a friend with the same problem told of the success he'd experienced with the herb. Eight months later, Janna reports that her episodes of dizziness are much fewer and farther between, though still severe when they do occur.

Hearing, sight, balance . . . The loss of one or more of these senses significantly diminishes the quality of life. Unfortunately, with age and sometimes for no discernible reason, we are robbed of our sight, our hearing, or our sense of balance. As we'll discuss later, taking ginkgo biloba extract, along with making lifestyle changes, perhaps under conventional treatment, can help you maintain and even strengthen your senses as you age.

THE GIFT OF SOUND AND BALANCE

The two main responsibilities of the ear are hearing and balance. Fed by thousands of tiny blood vessels that nourish all its cells, the ear has three main parts: the outer ear, middle ear, and inner ear. The outer ear—the part that we see—is composed of the pina or auricle (the folds of skin and cartilage) and the outer ear canal, which delivers sound to the middle ear. Within the outer ear canal are wax-producing glands and hairs that protect the middle ear.

The function of the middle ear is to deliver sound to the inner ear, where it is processed and sent via neurons to the brain. The middle ear is a small cavity within the eardrum on one side and the entrance to the inner ear on the other. Three small bones—the hammer, anvil, and stirrup—act like a system of angular levers to conduct sound vibrations into the inner ear. The hammer attaches to the lining of the eardrum, the anvil to the hammer, and the stirrup links the anvil to the opening of the inner ear.

A narrow tube, called the Eustachian tube, connects the middle ear to the throat. Ordinarily, the Eustachian tube stays closed, but it opens when we swallow or yawn in order to equalize air pressure within the middle ear and air pressure outside.

The inner ear contains the most important parts of the hearing and balance mechanisms. The vestibular labyrinth consists of elaborately formed canals, which are largely responsible for our sense of balance. The cochlea, which begins at the opening to the inner ear, curves into a shape that resembles a snail shell. When sound waves from the world outside strike the eardrum, it vibrates. These vibrations from the eardrum pass through the bones of the middle ear and into the inner ear. They are then disseminated into the cochlea, where they are converted into electrical impulses and sent to the brain by the auditory nerve.

The ear is a delicate organ, quite sensitive to injury, infection, and age-related degeneration. Hearing and balance disturbances can occur for many reasons, ranging from the simple and temporary (such as wax buildup in the ear canal or a viral infection that affects the fluid balance in the inner ear) to the more serious (such as a congenital defect in the structure of the ear or a traumatic and irreversible injury). Among the problems that ginkgo biloba appears to help are tinnitus (unexplained and chronic ringing of the ears), age-related hearing loss (connected to changes in the cochlea), and dizziness and vertigo. Let's take a look at what can go wrong and what we can do to protect ourselves from unnecessary damage.

Tinnitus

Tinnitus (pronounced "tin-it-tus") is any abnormal noise in the ear. It is an extremely common condition that affects nearly 36 million Americans. Tinnitus may be temporary or continuous, mildly annoying or extremely distracting. It can sound like a loud roar, a low hissing, or even a pulsating sound like the pulse of blood through a vessel (which, in fact, it often is). Some people with the condition describe hearing chirping, screeching, or even musical sounds. Tinnitus may occur in one or both ears. Most tinnitus results from damage to the inner ear or cochlea. There are many causes: A buildup of ear wax can cause tinnitus, as can a middle-ear infection, injuring the nerve that runs from the ear to the brain and central nervous system. Pulsatile tinnitus (the type that sounds like the beat of your pulse) can be caused by aneurysms and arteriosclerosis. Quite often, however, doctors can't identify the underlying cause.

Treatment of tinnitus depends on its cause (if it can be determined). If an ear infection is the problem, a doctor may prescribe antibiotics or other medications. Diuretics to eliminate excess fluid may be helpful in other cases. If you're particularly distressed about the problem, a sedative may be in order—and these drugs have also been shown to alleviate tinnitus itself, for reasons as yet poorly understood. Both acupuncture and chiropractic adjustments also have positive effects on tinnitus. In very rare cases, surgery to correct a structural defect may be helpful.

Often, however, doctors simply suggest that their patients with tinnitus simply try to block the sound with other sounds—for example, listen to the between-stations static on the radio, or play tapes of ocean or rainfall sounds. If tinnitus is related to hearing loss, being fitted with a proper hearing aid may help. Special hearing aids called "maskers" provide a band of masking noise that can alleviate high-pitched tinnitus unrelated to hearing loss.

Age-Related Hearing Loss

Hearing impairment is common among men and women over the age of 65. Indeed, some estimates indicate that more than one-third of people in this age group have a noticeable hearing loss. A particularly common, and usually severe, type of age-related hearing loss is presbycusis (from the Latin *presby,* meaning "old," and *cusis,* meaning "hearing"). Presbycusis usually begins between the ages of 40 and 50 and worsens progressively. The condition affects hearing in both ears, particularly the perception of high-pitched sounds.

This type of age-related hearing loss is often caused by changes in the cochlea or in nerves attached to it. Cells within the cochlea, the snail-shaped cavity in the inner ear, carry thousands of tiny hairs that convert sound vibrations into electrical signals, which are sent to the brain for processing. When changes in the cochlea take place, the signals are not transmitted as efficiently, resulting in hearing loss.

Unfortunately, there isn't much a doctor can do to reverse such age-related changes. Hearing aids, which amplify sounds as they enter the middle ear, can be extremely helpful in these cases. As you'll read later, taking GBE as both a preventive measure and to help improve your hearing may be effective as well.

Dizziness and Vertigo

The feeling of being light-headed or off balance is usually harmless and passes quickly. However, a type of dizziness called vertigo can be very uncomfortable, because nausea, vomiting, and ringing in the ears often accompany it. With vertigo, you have the sensation that you, or the area around you, is spinning, and spells can last for days.

Sometimes dizziness occurs and then disappears for no apparent reason. Inner-ear infections and the common cold can upset the balance in the inner ear, which may cause temporary dizziness and vertigo until the infection clears. Problems with circulation, which temporarily reduce the amount of blood getting to your brain, are sometimes the cause. Arteriosclerosis—the narrowing of vessels that carry blood to the brain—is often at the heart of the matter.

A special case of dizziness and vertigo is Ménière's disease, named for the French physician Prosper Ménière, who first described the condition in 1861. Ménière's disease is a disorder of the inner ear, which causes episodes of vertigo, ringing in the ears (tinnitus), a feeling of fullness or pressure in the ear, and fluctuating hearing loss. A Ménière's episode generally involves severe vertigo, imbalance, nausea, and vomiting. The average attack lasts two to four hours. Following a severe attack, most people find that they are exhausted and must sleep for hours.

An acute attack of Ménière's disease is believed to result from fluctuating pressure of the fluid within the inner ear. In some cases, the ducts may be narrowed from birth. Recent research focuses on a possible role of the immune system in attacking the healthy ear tissue, causing the imbalance through the inflammatory response.

Unfortunately, there is little your doctor can do for dizziness or vertigo unless it is caused by a treatable infection, in which case he or she can prescribe antibiotics to clear it up. There are also medications for Ménière's disease, including those that help reduce symptoms of nausea and dizziness. Sedatives are sometimes prescribed to relieve the severe anxiety that a serious attack can cause. Other treatments that seem to help some people include the use of diuretics and a low-salt diet to decrease the fluids in your body. Cutting down on the use of caffeine and nicotine may also help. Sometimes, eliminating food allergies can relieve symptoms of Ménière's disease.

Ginkgo Biloba and Your Ears

If you've been experiencing any hearing loss, tinnitus, or balance problems, the first thing you should do is see your doctor for a thorough evaluation. You'll want to find out, if possible, the root cause of your condition and receive any medical treatment available. You should also let your doctor know that you're interested in trying ginkgo biloba therapy so you and your doctor can work together to best treat your condition.

The good news is that ginkgo biloba extract, taken in standard doses of 120 mg a day, can relieve hearing loss and balance problems in most cases, most likely by improving circulation within the ear, in the connections between the ear and the brain, and within the brain itself. In addition, ginkgo's antioxidant and PAF-antagonizing properties not only help to prevent possible damage to hearing but may further clear the way for the body to heal on its own.

In a landmark study of GBE's effects on aging and the brain reported in the French journal *Presse Medicale* in 1986, researchers listed tinnitus as one of the symptoms GBE treats effectively. An earlier French study conducted in 1979 and published in a 1991 monograph titled *GBE: Pharmacological Activities and Clinical Applications,* reported that GBE was successful in treating 60 patients—35 men and 25 women—with hearing loss and/or vertigo and tinnitus. Half the patients were given 120 mg of GBE, while the others received a drug developed in Europe called nicergoline. The researchers reported that GBE was effective by all criteria, especially with respect to vertigo.

It appears, however, that GBE is most effective when the hearing or balance problem is relatively new and when the medication is taken for several months. In cases in which the hearing loss, tinnitus, or vertigo was prolonged, GBE's effects were far less pronounced. But it seems likely that GBE can *prevent* these problems from developing in the first place, thanks to its ability to protect cells from free-radical and other age-related damage, but this is as yet unconfirmed by scientific studies.

HEALTHY VISION AND AGING

Often compared to a complex, highly sensitive camera, the human eye is able to receive and transmit millions of disparate pieces of information in an instant, to make visual sense of a world filled with light, colors, textures, and images. As we age, and with certain degeneration conditions, the mechanisms in this sophisticated organ can become damaged and unable to transmit the messages the brain needs in order to assimilate and interpret images. Before we discuss a few of those conditions, and the way that taking GBE can help alleviate them, let's take a closer look at the eye itself, and how it allows us to see.

The structure of the eye is very complex, involving a long list of remarkable "devices" such as the cornea, pupil, iris, and lens—structures that focus and refract light and images until they reach the retina. Composed of 10 layers, the retina processes the light images projected from the cornea and lens. Rods within the retina perceive light, and cone cells perceive light and color. A small depression in the center of the retina, known as the fovea, provides the most acute vision. The small area surrounding the fovea is known as the macula lutea, and as a whole it is responsible for central vision. The retina is nourished by the choroid, a multilayered tissue composed of veins and arteries. The images received by the retina reach the brain by way of the optic nerve. The brain interprets these nerve impulses into what we perceive as sight.

When it comes to aging, there are two major problem sites for the eyes: the anterior chamber (located between the cornea and the iris), a space filled with a transparent fluid known as the aqueous humor. When something goes wrong here, a condition known as glaucoma results. Glaucoma is the leading cause of blindness in the United States.

The other problem area is the retina. Two different conditions may occur here: age-related macular degeneration and diabetic retinopathy. Studies indicate that GBE can help improve vision by helping the retina remain healthy. Let's take a look at these two common vision problems:

Age-Related Macular Degeneration

Sometimes known as senile macular degeneration, age-related macular degeneration (AMD) is the leading cause of severe vision loss in people over the age of 65. AMD involves the macula (which comes from the Latin word meaning "spot"), located in the central portion of the retina. The macula provides us with sight in the center of our field of vision. When we look directly at an object, the macula allows us to see the fine details. This sharp, straight-ahead vision is necessary for driving, reading, recognizing faces, and doing close work such as sewing or woodworking.

There are two forms of AMD: dry and wet. The dry form accounts for 90 percent of cases and is usually caused by aging and thinning of tissues of the macula. It often develops slowly and causes only mild vision loss.

Wet macular degeneration, on the other hand, is far more severe and rapidly causes vision loss. With the wet form of the disease, new blood vessels grow beneath the retina, where they leak fluid and blood and can create a large blind spot in the center of your visual field.

Certain factors are thought to aggravate or even accelerate AMD. These factors include high blood pressure, diabetes, and smoking. If you have high blood pressure or diabetes, talk to your doctor about the best ways to get these conditions under control. And if you smoke? You know the answer—quit right away and get some help if you need it. Conventional treatment for age-related macular degeneration is limited to laser surgery, which most doctors reserve for only the most severe cases of wet AMD. The laser beam destroys abnormal blood vessels. For milder cases, and for most cases of dry AMD, no other conventional treatment is available. (Later, you'll see how GBE may help improve vision in those with AMD, and help prevent the disease from developing in the first place.)

Diabetic Retinopathy

Those who suffer from diabetes mellitus—an endocrine disorder that prevents the body from metabolizing sugar properly—may experience vision loss, because high blood sugar levels can easily damage the delicate blood vessels of the eye. When retinal blood vessels bleed or leak, the retina swells and the leakage forms deposits on the retina. This condition is called diabetic retinopathy; eventually, the problem can cause serious vision loss.

Other forms of diabetic retinopathy include fluid collection in the macula, which may destroy your center of vision (as in AMD), and the growth of abnormal blood vessels on the retina, which may break or leak into the clear substance in the center of your eye, called the vitreous. This condition, called proliferative retinopathy, clouds the vitreous with blood so that light can't pass through to the retina. Scar tissue may also develop due to the abnormal blood vessel development, and this tissue may cause the retina to pull away from the back of the eye. Retinal detachment is an extremely serious condition that can lead to permanent blindness if it isn't treated immediately.

When allowed to progress too far, diabetic retinopathy may also be treated with laser photocoagulation, in which laser beams seal leaking blood vessels and inhibit abnormal blood vessel growth. In severe cases, including cases of retinal detachment, treatment may involve a vitrectomy, in which the clouded vitreous is completely removed and replaced with a clear solution. The procedure is often uncomfortable and may involve a period of recovery in which normal activities must be suspended for some time.

The best way to prevent or control the development of diabetic retinopathy is to manage your diabetes diligently, keeping your blood sugar under constant control. When diabetes is controlled, diabetic retinopathy is rarely a problem. If the condition becomes severe, laser surgery is an option you and your ophthalmologist may want to consider.

Ginkgo Biloba and Vision

First, if you suspect you may have a vision problem, see an ophthalmologist immediately. Diagnosing both AMD and diabetic retinopathy is fairly easy, and more treatment options exist the earlier you catch the disease. In addition to standard vision tests, your ophthalmologist may perform a fluorescein angiography. This process involves the injection of a yellow dye into your arm. The dye moves into your eye and into your retinal blood vessels. Then the back of your eye is photographed to determine if abnormal blood vessel growth and/or leakage have occurred (the dye makes the blood vessels easier to see in the photograph). The test may turn your skin yellow and your urine orange, but the condition is temporary and nothing to worry about.

Once you've received a diagnosis, you can start to take action. In addition to following your doctor's advice about treatment, you should consider taking GBE as well. Ginkgo's ability to fight free-radical damage and strengthen the smallest of capillaries may serve the potentially degenerating eye well. Ginkgo's general tendency to strengthen the modes of circulation, keeping the eye flushed with nutrients, may also contribute to keeping the macula strong and healthy.

As reported in *Ginkgo: A Practical Guide,* by Georges Halpern, M.D., German scientists in the early 1990s examined 25 people about 75 years of age. They found that those taking a dose of 160 mg per day showed improved vision within four weeks after the onset of treatment. The more damaged the tissue, the greater the effect—and without damaging healthy tissue. According to this small study, GBE appears to improve vision and improve circulation to the delicate and essential retina.

Animal studies of GBE also proved to be effective in reversing diabetic retinopathy—and probably for the same reason it works so well for AMD: By inhibiting free-radical damage, strengthening and toning the blood vessels of the eyes, and inhibiting excessive PAF production that might contribute to inflammation, GBE can help protect the eyes from damage due to diabetes, aging, and environmental factors.

You've now read about the remarkable effects GBE can have throughout your body—from your brain, to your heart, to your lungs and immune system, and now your eyes and ears—and indeed, the substance has a great deal to offer. Not only can it help treat and even reverse a wide variety of conditions, the herb may also help prevent many age-related, degenerative problems from developing in the first place.

Of course, as we've discussed, there is no miracle cure for aging. To age well, you'll have to put in some work yourself. In Chapter 8, we'll provide you with tips to help you stay as healthy as possible, for as long as possible, and to feel terrific while you're at it.

Find Out More About . . .

. . . Hearing and Balance Problems

Q. So far my hearing is just perfect, and I don't want to lose it as I get older. Besides taking ginkgo biloba, what should I be doing to keep my hearing healthy?

A. First, it's great that you're asking this question, and the good news is that there's plenty you can do to protect yourself. Here are a few tips:

- *Protect against sound damage.* Your ears interpret waves of varying air pressure as sound. These waves can produce sounds that are loud or soft and of high or low pitch. Very loud sounds, either sudden or chronic (such as those that occur in very noisy industrial workplaces) can damage hearing. If you work with or near heavy machinery or are bombarded by other continuous noise, protect yourself by wearing earplugs or earmuffs that bring most loud sounds down to acceptable levels.

- *Listen to music at moderate levels*—and teach your children to do the same. If you go to a loud rock concert, wear earplugs. If you use earphones to listen to music, keep the volume low.

- *Get regular checkups—especially if you work in a noisy environment.* Early detection of hearing loss will allow you to take precautions to prevent further damage—including taking GBE, which is more effective for early-stage than late-stage problems.

Q. This may be a silly question, but how can I tell if my mild hearing problem is caused by wax buildup?

A. The easiest thing to do is try a good ear cleaning, then see if your hearing problem resolves. However, never try to clean your own ears with cotton swabs or any other foreign object. The ear is extremely delicate and easily damaged. You might also push wax farther inside the ear, making your condition worse. There are good ear-cleaning kits that clean the ear with a safe chemical wash available at your local pharmacy. Follow directions carefully or ask your doctor to do it.

Q. I've had tinnitus and vertigo for many years, and am encouraged by ginkgo biloba's effects on these problems. I'm also interested in applying other alternative approaches to my problem. What can you recommend?

A. You may want to start taking a look at your diet. Cutting down on saturated fats and cholesterol, as well as addressing any food allergies or sensitivities you may have, are good places to start. A study published in the *Southern Medical Journal* in 1981 found a link between increased levels of lipids and Ménière's disease. More than 1,400 patients with inner-ear symptoms were placed on diets that decreased cholesterol and fat intake. In most patients, dizziness dissipated, feelings of pressure in the ears were alleviated, hearing improved, and the symptoms of tinnitus lessened in severity.

Much anecdotal evidence exists supporting the use of niacin and lecithin in combination to cure tinnitus, although large doses of niacin can be extremely dangerous, even fatal. A more popular natural "cure" is to take zinc supplements, but never take zinc with food or medication, because it can interfere with absorption of medicine and nutrients. Too much zinc may also be toxic. We suggest that you see an experienced nutritionist, as well as let your doctor know your plans, before taking more than the recommended daily dosage of any supplement.

. . . Your Eyes and Healthy Aging

Q. My father has diabetes and takes insulin. Can he take GBE?

A. Absolutely—unless he has a bleeding disorder or is taking a blood thinner or anticoagulant (like Coumadin) to treat another problem. In fact, GBE may help your father avoid some of the complications of diabetes, including diabetic retinopathy and arteriosclerosis, which, as you know, is a leading risk factor for heart disease, stroke, and other cardiovascular diseases.

Q. What is glaucoma? And could taking ginkgo biloba help prevent that condition from developing?

A. Glaucoma involves abnormal pressure in the anterior chamber, the space that contains the fluid called aqueous humor. Normally, this fluid circulates from behind the iris through the opening at the center of the eye (the pupil) and into the anterior chamber. Since the aqueous humor is produced constantly, it needs to drain constantly. The drain, located at the point that the iris and cornea meet, directs fluid into a channel that then leads it to a system of small veins outside the eye.

When this drainage system does not work properly, the fluid cannot drain and pressure builds up within the eye. Pressure also is exerted on another fluid in the eye, the vitreous humor behind the lens, which in turn presses on the retina. This pressure affects the fibers of the optic nerve, slowly damaging them.

Whether or not GBE can help prevent or treat glaucoma remains unknown. It is possible—though not proven or even studied—that by keeping the smallest veins in the eyes working efficiently, GBE can help drain the aqueous humor and thus reduce excess pressure on the retina and optic nerves.

Q. I want to protect my vision as I age. Apart from taking GBE, what can I do?

A. There are lots of things you can do to protect your vision starting by practicing eye safety. More than 40,000 Americans every year sustain eye injuries serious enough to warrant emergency-room treatment. Most of these accidents are sports-related, involving rackets, sticks, balls, bicycles, and pools. Gardening, sunbathing (excessive, direct sunlight can damage the retina), and do-it-yourself carpentry and other projects are other culprits. Simply wearing protective eyeglasses and sunglasses will go a long way in keeping your eyes healthy and your vision clear.

In addition to taking ginkgo, you can also help improve your vision with another herb. Called bilberry, this herb contains high amounts of proanthocyanidins, a type of flavonoid that protects the retina, and the eye itself, from the damage of aging. World War II British Royal Air Force pilots were given bilberry jam to eat, since it seemed to improve their visual acuity. You can also take bilberry in capsule, tincture, or tea form.

The other crucial thing you can do is to get regular eye exams. Experts differ about how often you should see an eye doctor, but healthy adults under age 40 should be examined about every three years, or more if they have specific vision problems. After age 40, you should see your eye doctor every year. Again, the more quickly you detect and treat vision problems, the less damage the disease process is likely to do.

CHAPTER 8

Healthy Aging: Body and Mind

A single substance that at once alleviates Alzheimer's disease, one of the most devastating and difficult-to-treat brain disorders; offers protection against cardiovascular disease, the nation's number-one killer; defends against and relieves allergies; lessens symptoms of premenstrual syndrome for women and impotence for men; and helps maintain vision, hearing, and balance even as we age. All without side effects or risks for the vast majority of people who take it.

Sounds too good to be true, doesn't it? Well, although ginkgo biloba extract certainly offers all of these benefits and more, it isn't the whole answer to any problem or to the general challenge of aging. Face it: There *is* no one answer, no magic bullet, no miracle cure for what ails you and the rest of us mortals living out the tail end of the twentieth century.

The good news is that we as a society appear to be making a return to a saner approach to health and medicine, one that combines the best of modern technology with both older healing traditions (including taking herbs like ginkgo biloba) and a new sense of responsibility and self-reliance. It is possible—even likely—that you will live to the ripe young age of 90 or 100 and, if you play your cards right, with a great deal of vigor, vitality, and strength.

But for that to be true, you're going to have to pitch in and do your part. Ginkgo biloba will help, as will some of the other well-known anti-aging substances now on the market that we'll discuss in Chapter 9. Taking advantage of the remarkable technological advances made in Western medicine during the last century, including diagnostic tests, medications, and surgical techniques, may also help extend your life. But the bulk of the work is up to you. And, since you're reading this book, we assume you already know that!

What are the secrets to longevity? Scientists all over the world are searching hard for that answer even as you read this. Chances are, they'll find what they're looking for not in their sophisticated, high-technology labs, but in the everyday lives of people who naturally live long healthy lives. According to the World Health Network, an Internet site for the study of aging and anti-aging, for instance, the cultures that live the longest include the Abkasians, who live on the eastern shores of the Black Sea in the Caucasus Mountains, and the Hunza, residents of the Himalayas of northern Peru. The Abkasians can claim 2,000 citizens who live to be more than 100, out of their population of just 150,000. They live simple lives, their stress levels are low, and their sleep cycles are longer and more natural. They work their bodies and minds throughout their long lives.

Studies have been done in this country, as well, about what helps Americans live longer. A landmark study performed in the 1980s by the University of Southern California School of Public Health found that seven specific healthy behaviors influenced mortality. They included: consuming only moderate amounts of alcohol; eating breakfast on a regular basis; maintaining a healthy weight; avoiding sugar and fat-laden snacks; getting regular exercise; enjoying seven to eight hours of sleep each night; never smoking cigarettes. On average, people who followed these guidelines lived about nine years longer than those with less healthy habits. More important, their quality of life at every age was significantly better than that of their peers.

In this chapter, we'll explore some of those habits in the context of the larger picture of what, for lack of a better term, we'll call a "healthy lifestyle." If you can make some or all of these suggestions habits, you can help yourself avoid developing the major diseases and disabilities associated with aging, including many of the ones we've discussed here: heart disease, stroke, memory problems and dementia, and age-related vision and hearing problems.

To us, a healthy lifestyle is one that offers you a sense of balance, a coherent but flexible structure, and a feeling of satisfaction—all while providing your body and mind with the nutrients, exercise, and rest they need to thrive. Here's how this breaks down.

- *Balance.* Within traditional Chinese medicine, health *is* balance—between yin and yang, heat and cold, dampness and dryness—and maintaining balance in all things internal and external is the ultimate goal for personal health and for the universe as a whole. We in the West tend to define the term almost as broadly: Random House Dictionary offers one definition of *balance* as "a state of stability, as of body or the emotions"; another refers to it as "a state of harmony."

When it comes to your health, maintaining balance in your diet, exercise, and emotional life is crucial. In today's fast-paced world, it's all too easy to overindulge in one area, sacrifice in another, and forget altogether what really makes you feel well, in control of your destiny, and satisfied. As long as you maintain this balance, you need not deny yourself the pleasure of a slice of rich chocolate cake or a whole day spent in bed reading, because you know that tomorrow you'll eat all of your vegetables and get yourself to your yoga class. Later, we'll show you how to add balance to your life as you develop healthy habits.

- *Structure.* Needless to say, late-twentieth-century life is not conducive to keeping regular schedules—meals are eaten on the run, exercise is crammed in on an occasional basis if at all, and any attempt to reduce stress or get enough sleep is met with dismissal and/or disbelief. By structuring your life so that you have the time to treat your body and mind well, by carving out specific times in which to take care of yourself, you'll be more likely to *enjoy* the pleasures of eating, exercising, and relaxing instead of resenting them.

- *Satisfaction.* Chances are, if you're reading a book about improving your health as you age, you have a strong desire to *live well,* not only live for a long time. To do so, it's important that you build the idea of attaining satisfaction, not only with your life in general but in your everyday activities. Enjoy the meals you eat, have fun while you are exercising. Set goals for yourself and then experience the satisfaction that comes from meeting them.

When you look back on those seven healthy habits that help men and women live longer, you'll see that they mirror this idea of balance, structure, and satisfaction: *moderate* alcohol intake, *regular* breakfasts, *routine* exercise, *restful* sleep, and simply staying away from toxic substances like cigarettes, fat, and sugar that disrupt the body's internal balance.

Creating a healthy lifestyle need not be complicated, and it certainly shouldn't be a stressful chore or something that leaves you feeling punished or bereft of pleasure. Instead, it should offer you a solid base of structure from which to work, play, love, dream, and grow old. When it comes to your health, that means establishing a healthy diet that provides you with all the necessary nutrients while satisfying your appetite, making vigorous and pleasurable exercise a part of your everyday life, and cultivating a comfortable and enriching mind-body connection through meditation or spirituality.

Before we provide you with some tips about establishing a balanced, structured, and satisfying lifestyle, we'd like to provide you with some encouragement: Men and women *are* living longer and healthier lives, and you can join that group starting today. Just read the following statistics:

The Healthy Aging of America

During the Roman Empire, the average life expectancy was just 22 years. In the United States, however, we've seen a constant increase: In 1850, the average American died at 45; in 1900 at 48; today it's 75.8, and people over the age of 85 constitute the fastest-growing segment of the population. Here are some other astounding statistics:

- In 1900, 75 percent of the population died before age 65.
- In 1990, more than 31 million Americans were over the age of 65, nearly double the number of people that age in 1960.
- By 2020, there will be more than 50 million older Americans.
- Every day, 10,000 more baby boomers celebrate their fiftieth birthday.
- According to the U.S. Census Bureau, a woman who reaches 50 years and remains free of cancer and heart disease can expect to live to her ninety-first birthday. An average healthy man who is 65 years old today will most likely live to see 81.
- More than 45 percent of people 85 years and older live independently at home; another 20 percent of this age group require help—but still live at home.
- The National Institutes of Health projects that by the year 2040 the average life expectancy will be 86 for men and 91.5 for women.
- In the year 2025, the number of Americans over 65 will outnumber teenagers by more than 2 to 1.

Think of it . . . tomorrow really does belong to you. By understanding the benefits of taking natural substances like ginkgo biloba, vitamins, and minerals, as well as by following a healthy lifestyle that helps you maintain balance and structure while enjoying your day-to-day life, your later years can indeed be "golden."

In the sections that follow, we offer you some tips on creating a healthy lifestyle by eating well, exercising regularly, reducing stress, and getting a good night's sleep, though clearly, it goes far beyond the scope of this book to give you all the information you'll need for this purpose.

EATING WELL

Nutrition is a complex and fascinating science, and, as you know from picking up the newspaper, we learn more about the impact of food we eat on our health every day. In essence, however, it's pretty simple: The human body requires about 40 essential nutrients in order to carry out its functions and maintain health. These nutrients include oxygen, water, protein, carbohydrates, fats, and a host of vitamins and minerals. Your body receives oxygen from the air you breathe; without it, you couldn't survive for more than a few minutes. Although most of us take oxygen for granted, study after study shows that the more oxygen you supply to your body's cells—by breathing deeply and circulating more oxygen-rich blood during exercise (and with help from ginkgo biloba!)—the better.

Water, which is found in most everything we eat and drink, is another substance we tend to take for granted. Water regulates body temperature, circulation, and excretion, and aids in digestion. It bathes virtually all of our cells in moisture. Nevertheless, few of us drink the eight glasses of water our body needs every day to stay in optimal health.

The other 38 or so essential nutrients are found in the food we eat. What we call a "balanced" diet is one that contains the appropriate amount—not too little, not too much—of those nutrients on a daily basis. In addition, a balanced diet involves providing the right amount of calories—the energy value of food—to maintain proper body weight. (A calorie represents the amount of energy the body would need to burn in order to use up that bit of food; any excess energy consumed is stored as fat.)

Within this general context, you have a vast number of choices to make every day about how you obtain these nutrients and how much you enjoy the meals you choose to eat. Here are a few suggestions we can make about establishing a healthy diet:

Balance Your Diet

Maintaining a balanced diet means more than simply giving your body its share of required nutrients. It also means having a healthy, balanced relationship to food. Here are some tips to get you started:

- *Follow the Pyramid Plan.* In the early 1990s, the United States Dietary Association (USDA) developed guidelines for a healthy diet. According to this plan, each day you should eat the following:
    —6 to 11 servings of complex carbohydrates (preferably whole-grain bread, cereal, and pasta, and brown rice)
    —2 to 4 servings of fruit
    —3 to 5 servings of vegetables
    —2 to 3 servings of protein (lean meat, fish, eggs, beans, nuts)
    —2 to 3 servings of low-fat dairy products (milk, yogurt, cheese)
    —Small amounts of fat and sugar

As we've mentioned in several of the chapters, you may want to bolster your intake of specific vitamins and minerals in order to help prevent or treat certain conditions: For instance, the antioxi-

dant vitamins and minerals are particularly important in the fight against cardiovascular disease and
cancer. You may want to consult your doctor and
or a qualified nutritionist about your specific needs
for nutrients and supplements.

- *Maintain a healthy weight.* Balance is the perfect
word to describe your need to maintain a weight
that's right for you: Not too thin, not too fat, but
just the right amount of weight to keep you feeling
well and strong. Without question, our society as a
whole tends to be fat: More than a third of all
Americans—men, women, and, tragically, children—are more than 20 percent over their ideal
weight. Appropriately, then, a great deal of attention is paid to cutting down on fat, sugar, and calories and boosting calorie expenditures by exercising
regularly.

However, when it comes to aging, a recent study
published in the April 1998 issue of the *American
Journal of Public Health* shows that weight *loss* is
far more unhealthy in those 65 and older than
weight gain. After controlling for a number of
clinical variables, including hypertension, diabetes,
and cardiovascular diseases, researchers found that
women with a body mass index (BMI) of 20 or
lower had a higher mortality rate than others.
Long-term weight change among study participants
showed that subjects who lost 10 percent or more
of their weight since age 50 had a relatively high
death rate—15.9 percent for women and 30.3 percent for men—over a five-year period.

Now, does this new study give you license to gain
weight indiscriminately no matter what your age?
Hardly. Before the age of 65, being overweight puts
you at risk for any number of diseases, including

cardiovascular disease, diabetes, and certain kinds of cancer. On the other hand, it does show that you need to be aware of your body's needs throughout the life cycle—and to pay attention to those needs. The time to start that process is now.

- *Consume all good things in moderation.* A varied diet is one that offers you the best chance of obtaining all of the vital nutrients you need as well as satisfying your desires and cravings.

Structure Your Mealtimes

Nothing interferes with a terrific resolution like eating well than a lack of routine. Eating on the run, forgetting to eat at all, neglecting the sense of community that comes from sharing meals with friends and family . . . these bad habits spell disaster for most people trying to establish a healthy relationship to food. Here are some tips to help you:

- *Establish a routine.* Let's start with breakfast. Remember, one of the top seven habits for longevity was eating breakfast—and when they said that, they didn't mean "every once in a while." They meant making breakfast a part of your daily routine. A morning meal that includes some protein and complex carbohydrates (such as a serving of low-fat yogurt with whole-grain cereal) will start your engines going with the right amount and kind of fuel.

    Once you've made breakfast a part of your routine, take a look at how you eat the rest of your meals. Could you manage to fit in a regular lunch hour for yourself, one in which you can take your time eating, take a little walk, and relax a bit before returning to your daily activities? Could you make dinner a family and friends event—at least once or twice a week on a regular schedule? The more you're able to do so, the better integrated healthy eating will become, no matter how busy and complicated your daily life tends to be.

- *Keep track.* If you have trouble with eating—if you eat too much of the wrong kinds of food, too little of the right kind, or simply have trouble focusing on the importance of diet—start keeping a food diary. Write down what you eat, when, and what you feel about eating it. That way, you may be able to get a handle on your daily eating habits and where they may need some work.

- *Plan and cook ahead of time.* Time has a way of flying by. If you make the effort to create a menu, shop, and even cook ahead of time, you'll be able to resist unhealthy temptations.

Satisfy Your Appetites

We can't emphasize this enough: Food is more than just a combination of nutrients; it should also provide you with pleasure and satisfaction. In order to make the most of your meals:

- *Be mindful.* Eat slowly. Too often we find ourselves gulping down food without really tasting its flavors or enjoying its textures and aromas. Then wait before eating more food than you might really want— it takes at least 20 minutes before your brain pushes the "satiety" button that tells your body that it no longer needs food.

- *Eat foods that leave you feeling healthy and well.* The substances in food—the vitamins, minerals, sugars, etc.—all have very specific effects on your body, and not all of them are beneficial. Pay attention to how you feel after you eat your meals. If you're often groggy and uncomfortable, or unsatisfied and tense, you may be eating too much, failing to eat a balanced diet, or consuming food that doesn't agree with your unique body makeup. Nutritious food, prepared well and eaten in a relaxed atmosphere, should nourish your body and your soul.

If you feel that your eating habits are really out of control, or if you want to refine your diet for specific reasons, we suggest that you visit a qualified nutritionist for more advice. No doubt he or she will add the following codicil: No matter how good your dietary habits are, your health will suffer unless you make exercise a regular part of your life. Read on. . . .

EXERCISING FOR LIFE

As we discussed in Chapter 4, the benefits of exercise are almost too numerous to mention. By making exercise a part of your life, you can help reduce your risks of heart disease, stroke, high blood pressure, some kinds of cancer, and myriad other diseases. It appears, too, that exercise can help you increase your longevity, probably by helping you combat the above-mentioned diseases as well as by reducing stress. According to a study performed by Dr. Xakellis of the University of Iowa College of Medicine, only about 9 percent of Americans over age 65 do some form of regular exercise. By starting now, you can make exercise part of your life before you get older. A study tracking the health and exercise habits of nearly 17,000 Harvard alumni found that men who burned at least 2,000 calories a week with exercise had a 28 percent lower death rate than men who exercised less or not at all.

Exercise is often perceived as a painful, tedious process, especially by those who need it most (i.e., those who participate in it least!). Properly performed, however, regular exercise soon becomes a positive, life-enhancing habit. It allows you to connect with your physical body in an intimate way, as you feel your muscles grow stronger, your heart beat harder, the tension of the day slip away. For many people, exercise is a time for the intellect to take a backseat to the physical body.

There are three basic components of an overall exercise plan, each one as important as the other. Here's a quick rundown:

- *Cardiovascular fitness.* Also known as "aerobic" exercise, the type of activity you need to perform to attain cardiovascular health involves increasing the intake of oxygen to the body. Aerobic exercise uses large muscle groups to get the heart pumping and the lungs filling with oxygen. With aerobic exercise, your body learns to burn fat more efficiently as fuel, a definite boon for people trying to lose excess weight. Among the best aerobic exercises are walking, jogging, aerobic dance, stair-climbing and step classes, cross-country skiing, rowing, and vigorous cycling. Without question, walking at a strong and steady pace is the easiest, safest, and healthiest way to get your heart pumping and your body burning more energy.
- *Strength training.* Strength training, also known as anaerobic exercise, is just as important to your

overall fitness as aerobic exercise. Muscle is more metabolically active than fat, which simply means that the body must burn more calories to feed and nourish muscle tissue than it would to maintain fat. Therefore, the more muscle you have, the more calories you'll burn every day.

• *Flexibility and balance.* Most Americans, even those who consider themselves to be in top physical condition, neglect flexibility. Part of the reason may lie in the noncompetitive nature of stretching: unlike aerobics and weight training, there are no times or weight limits to beat. Instead, stretching the muscles slowly and steadily to the limit and slightly beyond is an intensely personal effort, one that brings you closer to truly understanding the unique structure of your body. Practicing yoga is one of the best ways to attain a state of flexibility, balance, and coordination, and, fortunately, more and more local gyms and YMCAs are starting to offer classes.

It's important to note that exercise need not be demanding or elaborate to be effective. Moderate exercise—defined as thirty minutes a day of light activity such as walking and gardening—is almost as beneficial to one's health as higher levels of exercise. As you develop an exercise plan, keep in mind that people who learn to make exercise a habit in their lives also increase their self-esteem by setting and reaching new goals.

Balance Your Energy

To exercise or not to exercise; that is the question so many of us ask ourselves every day. Part of our resistance comes from the idea that exercise requires us to devote our entire lives to getting and staying in shape.

In fact, however, exercise should fit into your life in a natural and balanced way:

- *Exercise is not an all-or-nothing proposition.* There's no need to think that regular exercise means making every evening's aerobics class or running every single morning. If you can't manage these demands, so the thinking goes, there's no point in even trying. But don't let this approach stop you. Exercise can consist of a brisk walk to the market, an afternoon of gardening—even an hour of vigorous vacuuming!—any activity that requires your body to move and your mind to take a backseat to the task at hand.
- *Set realistic goals.* If you've been sedentary for a number of months or years, deciding to train for next month's marathon by running 10 miles every morning would be counterproductive and even dangerous to your health. After failing to meet the unrealistic goal, or straining your muscles trying to do so, you'd become frustrated and probably decide not to exercise at all. Set goals you know you can meet, or perhaps ones just slightly out of reach.
- *No pain, no gain is a myth.* Pain is a warning sign, a message from the body that something is wrong and needs attention. At the very least, if exercise causes you pain or leaves you feeling achy and sore, you're likely to end up discouraged and disappointed rather than stimulated. If you're just starting an exercise program, ask your doctor or a fitness instructor for some advice about setting appropriate limits.

Structure Your Activities

In the end, the ultimate goal is for you to make exercise a habit, not a chore or a dreaded and occasional assignment. You'll help yourself do this by following the tips below:

- *Schedule time to exercise.* For many people, exercise comes last on a long list of "things to do." Consider your exercise like a business appointment you've made with yourself, an appointment you can break only under very special circumstances.
- *Join a gym.* Many people find it easier to start exercising at a gym or health club. The support of fellow exercisers, the structure provided by taking classes, and the assistance from trained staff are often worth the price of admission.
- *Seek convenience and variety.* As you plan an exercise program, eliminate as many excuses as possible for not following through. If you join a health club that is open only during hours you're at work, for instance, you're obviously setting yourself up to fail. To alleviate boredom, you may want to alternate activities, taking a dance class one session, bicycling outside the next, performing yoga postures every other morning, etc. By varying your routine, you'll be more likely to keep it going.

Satisfy Body and Mind

Nothing sabotages an exercise plan faster than boredom and frustration. In order to maximize your potential for success, focus on the following:

- *Choose activities you enjoy.* Sounds obvious, doesn't it? But you'd be surprised at how often people decide to participate in a sport or activity not because they think it would be fun, but because of its purported health benefits. A week later, they've dropped the idea altogether. Try as many different activities as you can to increase your chances of finding the right activity for you.
- *Focus on the way you feel during and after you exercise.* Breathing deeply, working your muscles, and concentrating on meeting new challenges all add to the intensely personal experience of exercise.
- *Build self-esteem along with muscle.* Every time you make it to the gym for an exercise class, every mile you walk, every inch you lose in fat or gain in muscle will add to your sense of accomplishment and empowerment. Allow yourself to feel the pride that comes along with meeting each and every one of your goals.

After activity comes rest and recuperation—for your body and your mind. Few of us really appreciate how important it is to take time out to simply relax and let the stress and pressure of the day dissipate. In the next session, we'll give you some tips on how to reduce the amount of stress in your life.

REDUCING STRESS

As discussed earlier, stress is a difficult concept to define, mainly because each person describes what it feels like and how it affects him or her in a different way. Nevertheless, we do know that stress can have very negative effects on virtually every system in the body and contributes to the development or exacerbation of a wide variety of diseases and conditions.

Needless to say, one of the most effective ways of reducing the amount of stress you experience is by eliminating as many stress triggers from your life as possible: changing your job to one less fraught with tension, moving to a place more suited to your personality and taste, avoiding people who annoy you, etc. Unfortunately, making such changes is easier said than done, and will require some long-range planning and, no doubt, a good deal of self-examination.

Indeed, learning what is causing your life to be unbalanced—and what might help you make it more fulfilling—is the first step in the process of gaining control over your health. Many people find that the best way to get started is to join a support group of some kind, either one related to a specific health problem (like Weight Watchers or Alcoholics Anonymous) or one that focuses on a general subject of interest to you (a stamp-collecting club, or a church, synagogue, or other religious congregation, for instance).

In fact, more and more evidence exists that a social connection is an extremely important part of a healthy lifestyle. In a study published in the April 1998 issue of the *American Journal of Public Health,* a research team discovered a fascinating connection between healthy aging and religion. Over a period of 28 years, the researchers studied more than 5,200 people active in the Catholic, Protestant, Seventh-Day Adventist, Mormon, Fundamentalist, and other faiths. They found that those who were actively involved in religious organizations lived longer, healthier lives. More social contact, a longer marriage, more exercise, and a better likelihood of quitting smoking are a few of the other benefits of attending religious services frequently. The research team speculated that faith brings psychological benefits, and churchgoers often use faith as a coping mechanism and have a better support system for dealing with stress in their lives.

Learning to relax your body and mind—inside or outside of a community—will accomplish many health-related goals. It will reduce the time your body remains tense and in the "stress-reaction mode" and have a positive effect on your cardiovascular health. You'll learn that you have power and control over your internal environment—and maybe even your external one as well!

There are any number of stress-reduction methods, from deep breathing to meditation to biofeedback. Here we provide you with just a few ideas to get you started:

- *Yogic breathing.* Your breath or, more accurately, the respiration process, forms a link between your sympathetic (activating) nervous system and your parasympathetic (relaxing) nervous system. By learning to breathe deeply and regularly, you can help foster a healthy internal balance. Here's an exercise for you to try:

  1. Sit comfortably, making sure that your back is straight, your head is erect and facing forward, and your arms are relaxed.
  2. Close your eyes and attempt to concentrate only on your breathing. Let go of all other thoughts, just for these few moments.
  3. Visualize your lungs as consisting of three parts—a lower space located in your abdomen, the middle part just beneath your rib cage, and the upper space in your chest.

4. Breathe in through your nose, picturing as you do so the lower space filling first. Allow your abdomen to expand as air enters the space. Then visualize your middle space filling with energy, light, and air, and feel your waistline expand. Feel your chest and your upper back open up as air enters the area. The inhalation should take about five seconds.

5. When you feel your lungs are comfortably full, stop the movement and the intake of air.

6. Exhale in a controlled, smooth, continuous movement. Feel your chest, middle, and abdomen gently contract.

7. Make four complete inhalations and exhalations per minute, resting about two to three seconds between breaths. Rest for 20 seconds or so, then repeat the process until you feel more relaxed and in control.

- *Progressive relaxation.* Progressive relaxation is a technique used to induce nerve and muscle relaxation. Developed by Edmund Jacobsen, M.D., the technique involves tensing one muscle group and then relaxing it, slowly moving from one muscle group to another until every muscle group in the body relaxes. You can try it yourself by following this version of the exercise:

1. Stretch out on the floor with your knees bent and the small of your back touching the floor. If you like, support your head with a pillow.

2. Take a deep breath and tighten the muscles of your feet by clenching your toes.

3. As you relax your feet, exhale. Notice the difference in the way your feet feel.
4. Breathe in again, tensing the muscles of your calves. Hold the exertion for a few seconds, then let it go. Release the tension in your calves and in your mind.
5. Continue the process, tensing and then relaxing your knees, thighs, abdomen, chest, arms, shoulders, neck, and face. Each time you tighten and release the muscles, feel yourself sink into a deeper and deeper state of relaxation.

• *Biofeedback.* Biofeedback is one of the more "scientific" ways of exploring and utilizing the mind-body connection. Scientists developed biofeedback when studies showed that animals could control bodily functions once thought to be completely automatic by being given a reward or punishment. Physicians adapted those findings to design ways for humans to control unconscious functions through conscious thought.

Although there are several biofeedback methods—and you need to visit a trained professional to learn the technique—they all have three things in common: (1) they measure a physiological function (such as muscle tension or heart rate), (2) they convert this measurement to an understandable form (like a computer-generated graph or chart), and (3) they feed this information back to you. After practicing with the help of such a device, you may be able to learn to trigger your body to relax on your own.

• *Meditation.* Like biofeedback, meditation is a mental exercise that affects body processes. Meditation is performed for a host of reasons—religious, spiritual, and physical. When it comes to stress reduction, the purpose of meditation is to gain control over your thoughts so that you can focus on allowing stress to flow out of your body. Meditation for relaxation requires no special training, and can be done at any time of the day and in any comfortable space. We offer some helpful guides to get you started in the Resources section at the end of this book.

If meditation or other forms of stress reduction are new to you, you may find it very strange to have to "learn" to relax. But the fact remains that in today's fast-paced world, relaxation is considered a luxury, not the requirement for physical and mental health that it truly is. And once again, we can help get you started by emphasizing our paradigm of health: balance, structure, and satisfaction.

Balance Your Spirit

In addition to actively relaxing, you can help relieve stress just by having FUN! Indeed, just as we mentioned in connection with exercise, stress reduction should never be a chore but instead take place as an ordinary part of a balanced and healthy lifestyle.

- *Choose activities that stimulate as well as relax.* There's often a fine line between relaxation and lethargy. Lying around the house all day instead of getting outdoors and walking or taking care of relaxing chores like gardening or sewing may only lead to more stress. This is especially true when it comes to the all-American pastime of watching television. Although watching a favorite show or two may take your mind off the pressures of the day, studies have shown that the longer this passive activity lasts, the *less* relaxed it makes you feel. Instead of calming down, you become more irritable, guilty, and frustrated the longer you sit in front of the television. Reading, learning a new hobby, or even walking to a movie theater to catch the latest flick are much better choices.

- *Beware of high-risk behaviors.* Too many of us try to relieve stress and pressure by partaking in some rather unhealthy habits, such as smoking, drinking too much, or overeating. Although you may feel that these activities help to relax you, they are, in fact, increasing the stress on your body by forcing it to cope with the ill effects of these substances and behaviors.

Structure Times of Peace

- *Plan to relax.* Having enough time and energy to simply get through the day seems too much to ask for most of us. When you know a deadline is coming up or the week ahead is going to be particularly busy and stressful, try to schedule some time—even just a few minutes—every day to perform one of the relaxation methods described above or simply to take a walk to relieve the pressure.

Satisfy Your Spirit

Again, relaxation should never be a chore, but instead a release and a joy. These simple hints might work for you:

- *Create space.* Choose a room in your home, or at least carve out a space within a favorite room, to be your private area. Use it as a sanctuary from the confusion and chaos that surrounds it!
- *Increase your sense of self-esteem and control.* Learning that you have power and control over your internal environment and realizing that you can make successful positive changes in your physical and mental health will automatically raise your sense of self-esteem and give you a new sense of self-confidence.

Eating well, exercising regularly, and taking the time to relax are the keys to living a long and healthy life. Without doing so, you could take all of the ginkgo biloba supplements in the world and it wouldn't make any difference—or at least not enough of a difference—in your overall health or to your chances for living longer and better.

Taking it on faith that you understand your part of the bargain, we provide all the information you need to know about taking GBE and other anti-aging, health-promoting supplements in the next chapter.

Find Out More About . . .

. . . Aging

Q. Do scientists yet know why we age? Could we ever live forever?

A. There's no doubt that human beings are living longer than ever before, and we're making great strides in our efforts to live the second half of our lives with as much vigor and vitality as we did the first part. However, aging remains an essential fact of life for all living things, as does the final chapter of death. We struggle mightily against this inevitable consequence of life, but, as yet, we must eventually succumb.

Will there ever be a time when aging and death do not occur? Probably not. And as painful as the loss of loved ones and our former younger selves may be, we probably wouldn't really want it any other way. In a larger sense, we age and finally die in order to make room on this planet for the next generation of human beings to live and thrive.

However, scientists still don't completely understand, from a purely biological perspective, how and why we age. But they certainly have developed some pretty convincing and interesting theories. Here are just a few you may want to consider the next time you search for your next wrinkle or gray hair in the mirror:

• *DNA damage.* Each cell of the body contains DNA, the genetic blueprint that "tells" the cell how to behave and "who" it is within the body. Damage to the DNA, the genetic blueprint found within each cell, occurs continuously. While most damage is repaired, some cells remain defective. Some research suggests that the accumulation of these defects—which does not allow the cells and tissues to function efficiently—is the primary cause of aging.

• *Free radicals.* Free radicals, as you may remember, are unstable molecules. They attack the structure of cell membranes, creating metabolic waste products, which can darken the skin in certain spots (known as aging spots). They can also interfere with the synthesis of protein, which lowers our energy levels and prevents the body from building muscle mass. They disrupt cell metabolism, which could lead to cancer and other fatal illnesses. They also attack collagen and elastin, causing wrinkles.

• *Mitochondrial DNA.* This theory suggests that the loss of effectiveness of one of the cell's key components paves the way for age-related degenerative diseases. The mitochondria, which are the energy-producing bodies within a cell, appear to be particularly susceptible to free-radical damage. Once damaged, the cell loses its ability to produce energy and gradually dies.

• *Programmed cell death.* Experiments show that human cells will divide fewer than 100 times outside the body, and others show that there is an inverse correlation between the number of cell divisions and the age of the person from which the cells were taken. This theory suggests that the aging of cells is an active process, and even though they are unable to divide they continue to metabolize. As the cells gradually die off, the body dies.

• *Hormonal disruption and failure.* Another theory about the cause of aging centers on the endocrine system. Some scientists believe that an aging clock in the brain— probably in the hypothalamus—directly influences the slowdown in hormonal production. Among the essential hormones that diminish as we age are estrogen, testosterone, melatonin, and DHEA. In Chapter 9, we discuss the risks and benefits of the supplements now available to restore proper levels.

. . . Eating Well

Q. I've heard so much about soy products and how good they are for your general health and may even have anti-aging properties. What's the story?

A. High in protein, rich in vitamin B, calcium, and iron, soybeans are also the only food source that contains all eight of the amino acids necessary for humans to survive and stay healthy. They are free of cholesterol, low in saturated fat, and help lower blood cholesterol by interfering with the oxidation of LDL cholesterol.

  When it comes to helping you slow down the aging clock, soybeans contain antioxidants, which help fight against cancer and cardiovascular disease, as well as isoflavones, substances that act like estrogen in the body.

Q. Should I take more vitamin and mineral supplements as I get older?

A. That's a good question, and one that researchers at Tufts University recently answered with a resounding "Yes!" They found that people age 60 and over may require roughly a third more vitamins B_6 and D than young adults to maintain good nutrition. It could be that the elderly are unable to absorb and process essential nutrients as well as their younger counterparts. Another possibility is that the medications often prescribed in older Americans—particularly antihypertensive diuretics and anti-inflammatory agents—can inhibit the efficient breakdown and use of nutrients.

. . . Exercise

Q. I know that cardiovascular fitness is especially important to me, because heart disease runs in my family. I think I want to start with walking and then perhaps start cross-country skiing in the winter. What do I need to do to get started?

A. No matter what type of aerobic exercise you choose, you'll want to satisfy three basic criteria:

- *Intensity*. In order for exercise to have the maximum effect on the cardiovascular system, aerobic activity should be of a sufficient intensity, usually measured by the "target heart rate," or the rate at which your heart must work to provide health benefits to the cardiovascular system.

- *Duration*. Generally speaking, most experts recommend that a cardiovascular exercise session last between 30 and 40 minutes to provide maximum benefits, especially if you're trying to lose weight. When you first start to exercise, your muscles draw on quick sources of energy within their own cells, which can be obtained without increasing the body's supply of oxygen or burning fat. However, other research indicates that you can reap almost as many benefits by dividing your exercise up into three or more 10- or 15-minute sessions.

- *Frequency*. This one is key: To achieve lasting cardiovascular benefits, you must exercise on a regular basis. You should aim to exercise about three to five days per week, but don't get discouraged if you're not able to meet that schedule at first. Every time you move your body you're doing something positive for your health, and adding any habit to your life will take time.

Q. You mentioned exercising at my "target heart rate." How do I figure that out?

A. Your target heart rate is between 70 and 85 percent of your maximum heart rate. You can calculate your maximum heart rate by subtracting your age from 220. For the average 30-year-old, then, the maximum heart rate would be 220 − 40, or 190, and the target heart rate between 133 and 162 beats per minute.

Q. What about strength training? How should I get started?

A. Because the techniques of calisthenics and weight training are very precise and, if not performed properly, can lead to injury, we suggest that you visit a local gym or YMCA to receive personal instruction before you try to begin a program on your own. A weight-training routine should involve about 30 minutes of steady—but constant—stress on different muscles of the body using your own weight (i.e., push-ups, sit-ups, and other calisthenics exercises), free weights, or strength-training equipment (such as Nautilus or Cybex). You should formulate a specific routine with an exercise specialist.

. . . Stress Reduction

Q. Sitting still and trying to meditate seem to make me more anxious than relaxed. In fact, I feel like I'm about ready to jump out of my skin and I start to think about all of my problems past and present. Is something really wrong with me?

A. Not at all. You're simply not yet used to the feeling of "quiet" inside of your body and mind. It also sounds as if you might be resisting some of the deeper problems that come to light when you're alone with your spirit. The first thing you can try is adding exercise to your life—regular, strenuous exercise can help reduce some of the "antsiness" you feel when you're trying to meditate. You may simply need to burn off more physical energy before you're ready to relax. You may also need to more closely examine those problems—past and present—that crop up when you make room for them in your mind. The longer you avoid dealing with them, the more damage they'll do. Finally, don't give up on meditation. If you can't manage more than five minutes of quiet, focused time, then just do that much. Simply breathing deeply, concentrating only on your breath, will help relieve anxiety more than you might imagine.

CHAPTER 9

Using Ginkgo Biloba

Because you're reading this book, chances are you already know how easy it is to buy ginkgo biloba extract. Walk into any health food store, most pharmacies, and even some grocery stores, and you'll find a shelf (or two) of GBE supplements. Next to it, you'll probably find melatonin and DHEA, two other substances known for their anti-aging and other effects. And that's to say nothing of the dozens of vitamins, minerals, and other herbs readily available to consumers.

Without question—and as you've seen in the citations of study after study performed by eminent scientists at highly regarded universities and laboratories, and published in reputable medical journals—GBE is an age-old herb with some qualities that seem to be tailored to treat some very modern maladies. Indeed, the very diseases that plague us as we head into the twenty-first century—heart disease, allergies, and conditions related to the aging brain and senses—are the ones that the unique constituents of GBE act to prevent or reverse. And, as study after study to date indicates, it does so with very few, if any, side effects and at minimal cost.

As we discussed in Chapter 1, however, ginkgo biloba and its brethren so readily available in health food stores are powerful substances that you should take only with a great deal of care and knowledge, and with a certain amount of reserve. Again, as we've discussed before, research into GBE and other herbal and hormonal remedies continues in labs around the world, and even the most enthusiastic supporters of herbal medicine within the health care community offer a bit of caution with their support.

In this chapter, we'll discuss the current recommendations about purchasing and taking GBE, as well as how to become your own herbalist if you have access to fresh ginkgo leaves and nuts. In our question-and-answer section, we'll also briefly explore the other two most popular anti-aging "miracles," melatonin and DHEA. Before we do that, let's take care of the most important issue first: what makes up the GBE you find in health food stores, and who should NOT be taking it under any circumstances.

GINKGO BILOBA: THE EXTRACT

After gazing at a ginkgo biloba tree and examining its oddly shaped leaves, you might just wonder how it is that the unique qualities of this living thing become the capsule you take every morning and/or evening. Methods for making the standardized extract (which we describe in more depth later) vary, but all involve the same basic process. After harvesting the leaves—usually in the late summer, when their active compounds are at their greatest level—the herbalist dries them, then soaks them in a solvent of alcohol for a period of time to purify and distill the active compounds. Once in this form, the herbalist adjusts the remaining powder to the prescribed standard. He or she can then turn the powder into pills or capsules or, in the case of tinctures or liquid extracts, reconstitute it with water or alcohol.

When you buy GBE in any form, you want to purchase a brand that clearly states "Standardized" on the bottle. That way, you'll be more likely to obtain the correct amount of active compounds—specifically, the flavone glycosides (the antioxidants) and the terpene lactones (the substances that act on the blood and immune system response). According to the American Botanical Council, a dry extract of the ginkgo biloba leaf extracted with an acetone and water solution and then purified without the addition of any other substances contains the following: 22 to 27 percent flavone glycosides (mostly the antioxidants quercetin and kaempferol) and 5 to 7 percent terpene lactones (including ginkgolides A, B, and C, bilobalides, and ginkgolic acids).

In a standardized GBE formulation, the flavone glycosides make up 24 percent of the ginkgo biloba extract. As you may remember from Chapter 2, the unique flavonoids in ginkgo biloba play an important role in fighting against free-radical damage in the body. These substances tend to concentrate in organs containing a relatively large amount of connective tissue, including the heart, eyes, and lungs. In addition to their antioxidant qualities, they may also contribute to ginkgo biloba's ability to block platelet-activating factor (PAF) and thus reduce the inflammatory response and the blood's tendency to clot. The terpene lactones, including the ginkgolides A, B, and C and bilobalides, make up 6 percent of the standardized extract. They are what give the ginkgo leaves their bitter taste (which is why most people would rather take a pill than drink the tea!). No other plant contains these remarkable substances, which directly act to block PAF in the body. As such, they are largely responsible for ginkgo's ability to improve the circulation throughout the body and in the brain, which helps explain its therapeutic effects on such wide-ranging conditions as impotence, heart disease, and Alzheimer's disease.

Another substance related to the terpene lactones is ginkgolic acid, which is found naturally in the leaves and in the nuts of the ginkgo biloba tree. Manufacturers attempt to keep this substance at extremely low levels in standardized extracts, as the acid is considered toxic. Similar to a substance in poison ivy, ginkgolic acid in unstandardized products or in the dried leaves and nuts could theoretically cause adverse side effects, although no studies have actually documented any negative effects from the ingestion of ginkgolic acid. However, if you decide to cultivate and harvest your own leaves and nuts, it's important to do so with this warning in mind.

The FDA and Ginkgo Biloba

Now that you know how the GBE is made and what it contains, we have yet another warning for you: Not every brand of GBE offers standardized extracts. Some capsules merely contain ground-up ginkgo leaves, and probably aren't strong enough to have any effect. Others are created by the above process without the standardization steps. If you want to be taking the dosages used in scientific studies, you'll need to find supplements that are standardized.

But the warning doesn't stop there, either. As discussed in Chapter 1, ginkgo biloba and other herbal remedies do not fall under the purview of the regulatory agencies that control pharmaceuticals—namely, the federal Food and Drug Administration (FDA). The FDA supervises the development and marketing of all drugs sold in the United States, both prescription and over-the-counter medications. It is a branch of the Department of Health and Human Services, funded annually through the U.S. Congress, and has the authority to regulate food, drugs, cosmetics, and medical devices sold among the states or imported. The FDA is responsible for ensuring that these products are pure and unadulterated, and not misrepresented through false labeling, declarations of ingredients, or net-weight statements.

The FDA generally does not have jurisdiction over naturally occurring substances such as ginkgo biloba and other herbs, vitamins, minerals, amino acids, and certain hormones. Although that makes it easier and less expensive to attain these products, it also means that you cannot be positive that what you see is what you get. Although we know of no complaints about the quality of specific GBE brands, other forms of supplements have come under scrutiny for containing less than their stated active ingredients or for causing unwanted—and unproclaimed—side effects.

That said, it's important to note that the safety record for vitamin, mineral, and other natural supplements—including GBE, melatonin, and DHEA—has been consistently outstanding. According to summaries from the nation's poison-control centers, only one death was associated with the use of a nutritional supplement from 1983 to 1990, and that was due to the overuse of niacin by a mentally unstable individual. Prescription drug reactions or interactions, on the other hand, caused approximately 130,000 deaths *every year* during the same period. Nevertheless, you should remain responsible about your health: Continue to read current reports about the status of the supplements you take and visit a qualified herbalist or alternative medicine practitioner for professional advice.

Standard GBE: The Choices

Even standardized ginkgo biloba supplements are available in many forms and made by several different manufacturers. The following chart will give you an idea of what's out there, and provides you some insight into their specific qualities. Again, we suggest that you visit a qualified herbalist for advice before buying or taking GBE or other supplements.

Form of ginkgo biloba	Comments
Leaves you harvest yourself	This represents the purest, whole-herb form of the substance, but drying takes time and you might not like the taste of the tea. Also, you won't know how much of the active constituents you're actually getting. Best for long-term preventive health maintenance. May be more likely to cause side effects because certain undesirable substances—namely ginkgolic acids, found in a higher concentration in the seeds and nuts than the leaves

Form of ginkgo biloba	Comments
	and known to be somewhat toxic—are filtered out of standardized extracts but remain in the whole leaf.
Purchased dried leaves	Same as above, except there is the additional cost of purchasing the product.
Powdered leaves in pill or capsule form	Unstandardized, unprocessed whole herb, but usually not in enough quantity to have any effect. Avoid.
Organic unstandardized tinctures	Retains the benefits of the herb in its natural form, but the dosages aren't standardized, so you'll be unsure of how much of the active compounds you're ingesting.
Unstandardized capsules or pills	May be cheaper than standardized versions, but may still be highly processed. Again, you'll be unsure if you're getting what you pay for, and what your body will benefit from.
Standardized capsules, pills, or extracts—available in a variety of strengths (we've seen everything from 40 mg to 650 mg).	Supplement with standardized 24% ginkgo flavoglycosides and 6% terpene lactones—the ratios used in scientific studies. Also, some of the undesirable constituents in the whole leaf,

Form of ginkgo biloba	Comments
	such as ginkgolic acids—similar to compounds in poison ivy—are removed during the purification and standardization processes.
Ginkgo biloba mixed with other herbs and supposed nutrients in so-called "brain-enhancing" or "nutritional support" formulas	Ginkgo is often combined with other herbs—usually ginseng and gotu kola, which are thought to enhance intelligence and energy. Some supplements include vitamins, amino acids, and/or a variety of herbs. Some formulas mix ginkgo with substances that supposedly enhance absorption. Mixing ginkgo is fine as long as you know everything you are taking and in what dosage. Man of these supplements don't give you information on dosages of each individual herb. Avoid unless you're sure of what you're getting.
If you're in Europe, look for a ginkgo biloba/kola nut sparkling beverage containing 120 mg of GBE standardized to 24%.	Available in England, Germany, Spain, France, and Switzerland. We have no evidence of the medicinal efficacy of this product. Because it is mixed with apple juice, it is sure to be more palatable than plain ginkgo biloba tea.

GBE: The Dosage

Now that you know how GBE is made and what the standardized extract contains, no doubt you want to know exactly how much you should take and how often. Generally speaking, your dosage will depend on what you want to accomplish. To enhance general health, attain better mental clarity, and improve your circulation, we recommend that you take a total of 120 mg a day, either in three doses of a 40 mg capsule or two doses of a 60 mg capsule spaced throughout the day. For more serious problems, such as early-onset demintia, tinnitus, or other medical condition, you may want to increase the dosage to 40 mg four times a day or 60 mg three times a day for a total of 160 to 180 mg per day, after consulting with your health practitioner.

Although it is less convenient to take GBE in multiple doses, evidence suggests that the active constituents in GBE don't remain in the body for long; in fact, they peak about one hour after the administration of a dose. Some substances may concentrate in certain areas—particularly the brain, eyes, and ears—for longer periods. You'll maintain more consistent levels and enjoy better effects if you divide your daily intake of GBE into several doses. In addition, you'll want to take the herb consistently—every day—over a period of several months or longer in order to receive all of its benefits. Many people don't feel its effects until they've taken GBE supplements for four to six weeks. In the end, the longer and more consistently you take it, the better you'll feel and the more benefits you'll reap.

Tracking Medication Interactions and Side Effects

As discussed earlier, GBE acts as a blood thinner and anticoagulant, making it an excellent way to prevent and treat certain forms of heart disease and the group of conditions loosely termed "cerebral insufficiency" (which means not enough blood is getting to the brain for optimal health). That said, it's clear that the people who should NOT take GBE are those already taking a pharmaceutical blood thinner or anticoagulant. Such drugs include Coumadin (warfarin sodium), Streptase (streptokinase), Abbokinase (urokinase), and others. If you're unsure of what medications you're taking, talk to your doctor about it. If you are already taking aspirin for a heart condition, talk to your doctor about whether you can add ginkgo biloba to your regimen. In many cases, you may be able to do so, but if your doctor advises against it, we advise you to take his or her advice. Even when taking natural substances like vitamin E and garlic, both known to inhibit platelet stickiness, you need to exercise caution when adding ginkgo.

Apart from blood thinners and anticoagulants, no other drug has been shown to interfere with GBE's effects or, conversely, to be mitigated by GBE. In other words, you can probably take GBE with any other medication you're taking without risk. But we have to say this again: It's probably best for you to talk to your doctor and/or a qualified holistic practitioner if you're taking any medication or have a complicated medical situation. In addition, you probably should not take GBE if you're pregnant or nursing, since no studies have been performed showing the safety of GBE for newborns and infants. (On the other hand, there is no indication that doing so would harm you or your baby, but we recommend that you avoid taking substances that have not been thoroughly tested in this regard.)

Fortunately, the section on side effects will be quite short. In a very few cases, people experienced minor stomach problems when taking GBE, but these effects disappeared when treatment was stopped. In rare cases, people taking GBE reported developing headaches and dizziness; in most cases, ginkgo biloba actually improves these conditions.

However, if you should experience any of the following symptoms after taking GBE, see your doctor right away:

- nausea
- headache
- dizziness
- excessive bruising or bleeding from minor cuts
- bloodshot eyes

Again, although side effects are rare, widespread use of GBE in this country is fairly recent and much is yet to be learned about the substance and how it may affect certain individuals. In this and all things, it's better to be safe than sorry!

MAKING YOUR OWN GINKGO BILOBA

As discussed in Chapter 1, the remarkable substance we call ginkgo biloba extract is derived from a very common tree. Part of the family Ginkgoaceae, the order Ginkgoales, and the class Gymnospermae, the ginkgo tree is quite beautiful, with light green, fan-shaped leaves that darken throughout the summer, then turn a bright yellow before falling off in the autumn. Several varieties of ginkgo biloba trees have been cultivated; some have more erect shapes (*fastigiata*) than the standard, some have larger leaves (*macrophylla laciniata*), some have drooping branches (*pendula*), and some have leaves streaked with yellow (*variegata*). As far as we know, they all contain the same beneficial substances in their leaves and nuts.

Ginkgo trees grow slowly and don't produce flowers (on the "male" trees) or fruits (on the "female" trees) for at least 20 years, but they can live for up to 1,000 years. Cultivation takes patience, and growing ginkgo trees from seed won't yield impressive results for a long time—most 20-year-old trees are only about 20 feet high. You may be able to harvest a few leaves after only a year or so, but certainly not enough to keep you supplied with ginkgo biloba tea year round!

Fortunately, ginkgo trees line many streets and populate many parks around the country, and so it's possible for you to harvest leaves to make tea or the nuts to eat if you should care to do so. Even if you don't have a ginkgo biloba tree in your yard or neighborhood, a few herbal suppliers (including some on the Internet) can provide you with fresh, dried ginkgo biloba leaves at reasonable cost. It is best to consult with an herbalist or alternative practitioner about using fresh leaves in order to assure the safety of the resulting product.

What might be the advantages to buying unprocessed leaves? Many herbalists believe that using the whole herb, in its pure form, is better than using the standarized, purified extracts made in laboratories. In this form, you'll receive all of the plant's constituents, even those as yet unidentified or determined to have a specific health benefit—but which have an effect on the body.

To make a tea from ginkgo biloba leaves, you'll first

want to harvest them in the late summer, just before they begin to turn yellow and their active compounds are at their most plentiful. Dry them in a cool, dry place (out of the sun), then store them wrapped in paper, then in plastic, away from light and heat.

To make the tea, finely crush about an ounce of dried leaves into a non-aluminum teapot, cover with about a pint of water, and simmer for five minutes. Remove the pot from the heat, allow the tea to steep for 10 minutes, strain, and enjoy. If you're like most people, you may find that the tea has an unpleasantly bitter taste. Try adding honey, lemon, or palatable herbs such as peppermint for a more pleasant brew.

Ginkgo Nuts

Although we in the West have concentrated on the healing properties of ginkgo biloba leaves, Chinese herbalists use three parts of the ginkgo biloba tree as medicine—the nuts (also called the fruit), the seeds, and the leaves. They carefully prepare them by boiling them for some time, then add the nuts and seeds to soups as medication for alleviating "wet" conditions such as asthma and chronic diarrhea.

However, we don't recommend that you try to use other parts of the tree yourself. The nuts and seeds contain terpene lactones called ginkgolic acids that irritate the skin. In fact, contact with the ginkgo nut, a plumlike fruit that matures in late autumn, can cause skin rashes. Swallowing even a small piece of the raw nut or its seeds can result in painful spasms. Fortunately for those with an adventurous appetite, ginkgo nuts are often available in health food stores, herbal stores, or Chinese grocery stores. Once purified through boiling and other methods, ginkgo nuts are nutritious, high in protein, and low in fat.

Now that you've read all about GBE and its known effects on the body, it's up to you to make an educated decision about whether or not the herb is right for you. By all accounts, GBE appears to be one of the most healthful and safe herbs currently available. In the Appendixes that follow, we provide you with a list of resources to help you find out more about GBE and other topics we've discovered in this book, plus an herbal guide to help you find other natural remedies for the conditions we've discussed in this book. And just for fun, we've added a section on improving your memory and even using GBE to help keep your pets healthy!

Find Out More About . . .

. . . Taking GBE

Q. I'm a healthy 50-year-old man who wants to take GBE because heart disease runs in my family. I take no other medication, but my doctor doesn't want me to try it because he doesn't know anything about GBE or other herbs. What should I do?

A. That's a question without an easy answer. Many conventional physicians who are reputable and highly qualified find it difficult to accept the tenets of herbal medicine or other alternatives. You should discuss the matter thoroughly with your doctor—and bring him this book if he'd like more information—to make absolutely certain that there is nothing in your medical history or current status that might indicate that GBE would not be helpful for you. If you continue to meet strong resistance and feel uncom-

fortable about it, you may want to consider changing doctors—especially if you're considering exploring other alternatives as well. This is hardly a matter to take lightly,
especially if you've been a patient of this doctor for a long
time. Nevertheless, striving for health and vitality in this
complex world is not an easy proposition, and you need all
the support you can get.

Q. Can I take ginkgo biloba supplements every day for the
rest of my life?

A. So far, no evidence has suggested any toxicity or adverse
effects with long-term use. In fact, long-term use is more
likely to produce the desired effects, because levels of the
active properties in ginkgo biloba will reamin constant.

Q. I bought a brand of GBE that combined ginkgo biloba with
ginseng and gotu kola. Can you tell me what these other
herbs are and what they do in the body?

A. Grown in China and in the northeastern United States, ginseng has been used in Chinese medicine for centuries. Ginseng is now a popular herbal remedy in the West, particularly known for its energy-enhancing properties. Gotu kola
is a plant traditionally used in India as an herbal antibiotic,
nerve tonic, and in the treatment of such mental disorders
as epilepsy, schizophrenia, and memory loss. Gotu kola is
thought to enhance intelligence and energy, and is a good
anti-inflammatory. Gotu kola is not a kola nut (used to
make cola drinks) and, unlike the kola nut, doesn't contain
caffeine. For more information about ginseng and gotu
kola, see Appendix 2.

. . . Buying and Using Supplements

Q. I'm still concerned about the quality of the supplements I buy at the health food store. Is there any way I can be absolutely sure of what I'm getting?

A. Unfortunately, no. Because phytomedicines, or herbal medicines, aren't regulated in the United States, buying and using them is usually a case of "buyer beware." The best way to ensure that you are getting a high-quality supplement is either to talk to an experienced herbalist about brands she or he knows are good, or to make inquiries to the company that manufactures your product to get a sense of their commitment to holistic health, their company practices, and their level of knowledge. In other words, do your research and talk to someone who has done his or her own!

Q. I've heard a lot about melatonin. What exactly is melatonin and what is it supposed to do?

A. Melatonin is a hormone secreted by the pineal gland, a tiny, pinecone-shaped endocrine gland located at the base of the brain. Nicknamed the "chemical expression of darkness," melatonin is produced almost exclusively at night. It acts as a sleep promoter and is apparently a key to maintaining the body's circadian rhythms—the daily fluctuations of hormones and other body processes, including the sleep/wake cycle. Indeed, melatonin is best known as an effective sleep aid: Taken about an hour before bedtime in strengths as low as 0.3 mg, melatonin can help ready the body and the mind for a restful night's sleep.

In addition, recent research indicates that melatonin also acts as a powerful anti-aging, health-promoting substance in the body by acting as a:

- *Master hormone.* Melatonin may trigger the release or suppression of other hormones. For instance, the blood level of melatonin appears to trigger the adrenal glands and gonads to increase or suppress the secretion of female and male sex hormones—signaling the beginning of puberty and the onset of menopause in women.
- *Immune system booster.* Melatonin apparently stimulates the production of antibodies, the body's first line of defense against infection. It also restores production of natural killer cells, a critical part of the immune system that appears to decline with age.
- *Super antioxidant.* Like GBE, melatonin may act as an effective weapon against free radicals, which, as you've read, are associated with a myriad of health-related diseases, including arteriosclerosis and cancer.

Q. Is melatonin safe to take?

A. To date, no serious side effects or drug interactions have been noted with melatonin—and that's after years of research among thousands of study participants and the use of the hormone among hundreds of thousands of consumers. However—and this is a big however—melatonin is a powerful body chemical that affects wide-ranging changes in the body. No one knows exactly how much of the substance an individual should take or what the long-range effects of adding a hormone to the body will be. Melatonin and DHEA (discussed below) appear to stimulate the release of IGF-1, a substance responsible for the growth of cells through the body—cells that may be cancer cells. Although no studies to date show a direct connection between taking melatonin or DHEA supplements and cancer, there exists the potential that taking too much of these hormones will exacerbate the development of certain cancers. Keep reading, and stay alert to new reports about its safety and efficacy.

Q. I heard about a harmful sleeping remedy sold in health food stores. Is it related to melatonin?

A. You may be talking about a dietary supplement, known as Sleeping Buddha, sold in health food stores for a short period of time in early 1998. It is not related to melatonin. The FDA became involved with the substance after the agency discovered that it contained a prescription-strength sedative called estazolam that could cause serious side effects in some individuals. In particular, estazolam can damage unborn children and so should never be taken by pregnant women. The Canadian manufacturer of the substance began a voluntary recall of all the Sleeping Buddha products distributed in the United States.

Q. I've heard about DHEA and its anti-aging properties. Is this another hormone?

A. Yes. Short for dehydroepiandrosterone, DHEA is a steroid hormone produced by the adrenal glands as well as by certain skin and brain cells. During the mid-1980s, scientists discovered that levels of natural DHEA decrease as we age, so that by the time we reach our 80s, we have just 15 percent of our youthful levels. They also linked DHEA to a wide range of essential body processes that decline as we age. The theory is that replacing the DHEA we lose as we age will help restore certain functions. Studies show that DHEA helps to incrase the libido and general vitality, lower risk of heart disease, and even reverse present cardiovascular damage, diminish the effects of Alzheimer's disease and other degenerative brain disorders, and boost the immune system.

However, taking DHEA is not without risk. Because DHEA is a steroid hormone, it can cause unpleasant side effects, including acne, unwanted hair growth, deepening of the voice, irritability or mood changes, insomnia, and fatigue. And, as discussed previously, DHEA stimulates the release of a growth factor that could potentially be connected to the spread of certain cancers.

Appendix 1

The Healing Herbs A–Z

Ginkgo biloba is only one of hundreds of herbs used as medicine here in the United States and around the world. In many of the chapters you've just read, we've recommended other herbs to treat certain conditions or simply as healthful additions to a healthy lifestyle. Now we describe those herbs in more depth, as well as mention others that you may find helpful and why.

For the most part, you can use ginkgo biloba extract in combination with any of the herbs we list here. Please be aware, however, that although herbs tend to work in a more gentle and safe way upon the body, they also have powerful effects—especially if you're also taking modern pharmaceuticals that work on the same organs or systems. We urge you to visit a qualified herbalist or alternative medicine practitioner for advice about the safest and most beneficial ways to use herbs to improve and maintain your health.

Aloe (Aloe vera)

Otherwise known as Lily of the Desert, the aloe vera plant originally grew in the tropics of Africa, where the gelatinous inside of the plant leaves was applied as an antiseptic to promote the healing of tropical wounds. Aloe is one of the oldest and most effective of the therapeutic herbs. The inner mucus of the leaf consists of over 200 nutrients and works as an antifungal as well as a coagulant in the treatment of skin abrasions. Aloe has even been used to combat the HIV virus; holistic medicine has recently turned to the use of aloe as a viral inhibitor, buffering healthy cells against the virus.

Sold in the form of a cosmetic gel, aloe is widely used for the skin as a moisturizer, a pH balancer, and a skin softener. The aloe gel, also available in an ointment, prevents infection and treats burns, eczema, and ringworm. As a powder or powder capsule, aloe is taken as a sedative and as a digestive aid. Aloe leaves are known to stimulate the flow of bile, absorb toxins, and to generally promote the growth of healthy colon bacteria. Prepared in a tincture, aloe relieves constipation and stimulates the appetite. Since it does have a purgative effect, aloe is not recommended to women during pregnancy.

Butcher's Broom (Ruscus aculeatus)

For centuries Mediterranean butchers used the stiff, leavelike twigs of this plant to sweep off scraps of meat from the cutting block, whereas the root of the plant was boiled and drunk as an anti-inflammatory agent. Today the herb is very popular with European women who use its extract in capsule form to prevent and shrink varicose veins. Saponins, the plant's active chemical component, are known to constrict veins and decrease the permeability of capillaries, making butcher's broom a beneficial aid to the circulation of blood in the hands and feet.

Cayenne *(Capsicum frutescens)*

This red hot chili pepper, supposedly brought from India to the West by Christopher Columbus, is an effective stimulant of the digestive and circulatory systems. The fruit of the cayenne pepper produces HCL, increasing the body's ability to digest, and influences the flow of digestive glandular secretions. It increases liver enzymes and thermogenesis, effective in the processes of fat metabolism and weight loss; heals intestinal ulcers; and removes, cleans, and rebuilds stomach tissues. As a circulatory aid, it increases and equalizes blood circulation (to prevent strokes and heart attacks), and heals ulcers in the cells of arteries, veins, and capillaries.

In the form of a powder, cayenne can be rubbed on toothaches to minimize pain. As a cream or massage oil, the extract of cayenne can offer relief from arthritis and rheumatism. When the fruit is prepared as a tincture or infusion, it best stimulates circulation and digestion. However, the seeds of the plant are toxic and the skin of this fruit can be irritable to the skin and eyes, so handle with care. Cayenne is not recommended during pregnancy, and excessive consumption can lead to gastoenteritis and liver damage.

Chamomile *(Chamaemelum nobile)*

Since the dawn of history Germans have used this sweet, fruity-smelling plant, dubbed by the ancient Greeks as "ground apple," as an aid to digestive and menstrual disorders. The chemical bisabolol, contained in the plant's leaves and flowers, acts as a general muscle relaxant and mild sedative, which explains why a cup of chamomile tea works as a perfect natural sleep aid and anxiety reducer.

Teas, tablets, and tinctures made of chamomile flowers soothe menstrual cramps and relax the smooth muscles that line the digestive tract, preventing vomiting and offering relief from irritable bowel syndrome and indigestion. As an anti-inflammatory agent and an anti-allergen, chamomile is now a common ingredient in hair and skin care products and can be applied as an ointment to treat insect bites and minor skin irritations. Persons sensitive to ragweed may experience allergic reactions to chamomile, and because it may act as a uterine stimulant, the use of chamomile oil is not advised for women during pregnancy.

Dandelion

Rich in vitamins A and C and high in minerals, the dandelion is much more than a common yard nuisance. The root of this flower promotes overall health of the digestive system, acting as a natural diuretic, inducing regularity, and ridding the body of excess salt and water. Rich in lecithin, dandelion root enhances liver and gallbladder functioning, prevents the formation of gallstones, and is believed to protect the liver against cirrhosis. Dandelion's high concentration of potassium prevents iron deficiency, reduces high blood pressure, regulates fluids, and normalizes the heartbeat.

Though readily available in capsules, dandelions are often boiled and chilled, added to salads, or eaten hot as greens. Dried and powdered, dandelion can be added to beverages such as tea or coffee for nutritional value and digestive purposes.

Dong Quai *(Angelica sinensis)*

Commonly referred to as tang-kuei, this plant is very popular in China and Japan to treat dysmenorrhea and ailments affecting the female reproductive organs and muscles of the uterus. Known as the woman's herb, dong quai regulates the menstrual cycle and provides hormonal balance. The root of this plant is commonly given to women after childbirth as an antibiotic, pain reliever, and blood purifier, as well as to women suffering from symptoms of PMS and menopause, including depression, nervousness, abdominal cramping, hot flashes, and vaginal dryness.

Dong quai is most commonly sold in the form of powder capsules and is not recommended for pregnant women.

Echinacea *(Echinacea angustifolia)*

Echinacea, "King of the Blood Purifiers," derives from the purple coneflower. The root and rhizome of this flower were used by Native Americans as an antibiotic and as a blood detoxifier in cases of snakebites. Echinacea is most popular today in the prevention of flus, common colds, mouth and gum inflammations, and prostate irritations. Recent studies conclude that the fatty acids, polysaccharides, and glycosides found in the root of the herb immensely stimulate and strengthen the immune system, increase resistance to infection and virus, and suppress tumor production. As a result, echinacea is currently being administered to AIDS patients to stimulate T-cell production and to persons receiving chemotherapy as a means to restore normal immune function.

Echinacea is most commonly taken in the form of powder or capsules and is beneficial to pregnant women as an effective immune stimulant, although excessive comsumption can lead to dizziness and nausea.

Feverfew (Chrysanthemum parthenium)

Otherwise known as bachelor's button or featherfew, the leaves of this plant have been used since the Middle Ages as a fever reducer. Today feverfew is primarily used to alleviate and prevent migraine headaches, but it also works to restore normal liver function and decongest the lungs and bronchial tubes. Since its leaves are extremely bitter, it is taken in pill or capsule form and is not recommended for children under two years of age.

Garlic (Allium sativum)

Ancient Egyptians, Greeks, and Romans have used garlic cloves for thousands of years as a cancer treatment, yet only recently has garlic been seriously researched by scientists for its antioxidant and anti-tumor properties. As an allium oil and sulfur compound, garlic is believed to inhibit cancer cell formation, suppress tumor formation, and modulate the metabolism of carcinogens. Studies have also concluded that garlic protects the body against the effects of radiation and the liver from damage induced by synthetic drugs and chemicals used in cancer treatments. Garlic is beneficial for the circulatory system and for maintaining good cardiovascular health; it acts as an anticoagulant, reduces blood cholesterol levels (while increasing HDL, "good cholesterol" levels), and lowers blood pressure. By lowering blood sugar levels, garlic also reduces the risk of late-onset diabetes.

Garlic can be taken as fresh cloves in salads or juices, or as oil capsules or pearls. Taking too much garlic can irritate the stomach and cause heartburn. Doctors warn that doses of more than ten cloves a day can be toxic. Because garlic can cause colic in infants, it is not recommended for women during pregnancy or lactation.

Ginseng

Though there are three different types of ginseng—Chinese (*P. ginseng*), American (*P. quinquefolius*), and Siberian (pseudo ginseng or *E. sentocosus*)—all three forms are known for their rejuvenating properties. Germanium, found in the root of the plant, provides energy to the body, promotes regeneration from stress and fatigue, and improves memory and general brain functioning. Since the days of ancient Greece, ginseng has also been used as an aphrodisiac, due to its ability to heal prostrate disorders and promote male hormone production.

Ginseng is commonly taken in the form of tea, root powder, capsule, or tablet, but since it acts as a stimulant, do not combine it with the use of other stimulants such as coffee, cola, or caffeinated tea. Ginseng produces testosterone and is therefore not recommended for long-term use by women. Follow dosage carefully.

Goldenseal *(Hydrastis canadensis)*

Cherokee Indians in the Northeast of the United States introduced the use of goldenseal root as an antibacterial and antacid. Hydrazine, the active ingredient in the plant's root, is primarily used as an immune stimulant and decongestant, effectively reducing the inflammation of mucous membranes and preventing respiratory infections. Goldenseal raises low blood pressure, and as a digestive and bile stimulant, it relieves chronic gastritis and enteritis, improving the digestive process and maintaining healthy liver functioning. This herb is recommended for infections or inflammations of the uterus, urethra, and vagina and can also prevent morning sickness in pregnant women and reduce symptoms of PMS.

Since the goldenseal plant should not be eaten fresh, the plant's root is often powdered and sold as a compound tablet or capsule. It can be used in eardrops for wax buildup (but not in the case of perforated eardrums), in mouthwash and gargles (for gum inflammations and mouth ulcers), and in a douche for yeast infections. This herb is not recommended for pregnant women or for persons with high blood pressure.

Green Tea (various spp.)

Modern science is finding new benefits from the Far East's most popular and ancient beverage—green tea. With twice the catechins (tea's active ingredient) of black tea, green tea has been linked to reduced cases of pancreatic and stomach cancers in areas of the Far East with the highest percentage of green tea consumption. It is believed that the antioxidant catechins in green tea destroy free radicals and therefore protect the body against cancerous tumor development. These studies have also found the tea to contain antiviral properties that enhance the immune system and destroy bacteria. Green tea is considered vital to metabolism and is favored in the treatment of dysentery and rheumatism.

Lavender *(Lavandula spp.)*

The highly aromatic character of its flower has made lavender one of the most popular herbs since ancient times. Arab and European cultures have used the antiseptic, antibacterial, and carminative properties of the herb to heal topical wounds, relieve indigestion, and to stimulate the circulatory system.

The essential oil extracted from lavender flowers treats insect bites and stings. As a hair rinse it expels nits and lice, and in mouthwash lavender fights halitosis. The most common use of lavender leaves is as an infusion to treat nervousness, exhaustion, tension headaches, and digestion problems.

Licorice *(Glycyrrhiza glabra)*

As one of China's most popular healing herbs, licorice has been used since 500 B.C. as a general detoxifier and treatment of stomach ulcers. Recent studies have found that glycyrrhizic acid, found in the root of the licorice plant, stimulates the production of interferon—the body's own antiviral compound and immunal stimulant—arming the body against immune deficiency diseases and viral infections such as herpes and herpes simplex. Licorice is anti-inflammatory, soothing gastric mucous membranes and chest congestion, stimulates adrenal function, and helps to raise blood sugar levels to normal, improving the body's ability to handle stress. Licorice root is also used to normalize ovulation in women experiencing infrequent menstruation.

Licorice root does cause fluid retention and is not recommended for persons with high blood pressure or persons taking digoxin-based drugs.

Meadowsweet *(Filipendula ulmaria)*

Owing to the refreshing and sweet aroma of its flowers, meadowsweet was a popular air freshener in the Middle Ages and is reportedly one of Queen Elizabeth's favorite scents. The synthetic form of meadowsweet is acetylsalicylate, more commonly known as aspirin. The leaves and flower tops of this plant reduce fever and relieve pain and inflammation, but unlike aspirin it does not cause gastric ulceration and bleeding if taken over long periods of time.

Meadowsweet is usually dried for an infusion or tea and taken to relieve symptoms related to the common cold, rheumatic pain, and upset stomach. It can also be used in a tincture for gastric ulcers or in a compress for arthritis pain. Meadowsweet should be avoided in cases of salicylate sensitivity.

Papaya *(Carica papaya)*

The fruit of the papaya tree, abundant in Hawaii, where they are referred to as "medicine trees," is primarily recognized as a digestive aid. The fruit contains papain—chemically similar in structure to the synthetic antacid pepsin. But while synthetic antacids eventually cause the stomach to produce more acid, not less, resulting in more gastrointestinal disturbance, papaya juice, tablets or dried fruit relieves indigestion naturally and safely by breaking down proteins and stimulating metabolic activity and digestion. Less commonly known, the papaya is also an effective external treatment for hemorrhoid irritation.

Peppermint *(Mentha piperita)*

Although cultivated by the ancient Egyptians, peppermint has been an integral part of Chinese medicine since A.D. 659. Herbalists use the leaves, stem, and essential oil of the peppermint plant, which is primarily known as a relaxant for the lower sphincter muscle and esophagus. As a digestive aid, peppermint tea stimulates the flow of digestive fluid in the stomach and alleviates intestinal problems, nausea, and diarrhea. Currently peppermint is used in the treatment of irritable bowel syndrome, colitis, and Crohn's disease. Peppermint is also extremely energizing; it acts as a nerve stimulant and oxygenates the blood. Peppermint leaves are usually dried for tea, but when added to an enema it can relieve colon discomfort.

Rosemary *(Rosmarinus officinalis)*

Ancient Greeks believed that the rosemary plant strengthened memory, and recent studies suggest that the plant may be a preventative agent for breast cancer. Thought of as an all-around stimulant and antioxidant, rosemary is a strong brain function and memory enhancer—sharpening the senses and alleviating nervous ailments. As blood cleanser, it benefits capillary circulation, bringing more blood to cells and strengthening the heart.

Rosemary oil is often poured in baths for aching limbs and exhaustion, added to hair for follicle strength and dandruff control, and added to massage oils to soothe muscle tension. A drop of rosemary on the pillow is an effective way to fight insomnia. The ground leaf (usually in capsules or infusions) acts as an antidepressant and digestive aid. Rosemary is a compress relieves rheumatic pains and sprains.

St. John's wort *(Hypericum perforatum)*

During the Crusades this healing herb was named for the Knights of St. John's of Jerusalem, who used it to treat wounds on the battlefield. The flowers of this plant have astringent, analgesic, and anti-inflammatory properties, which make it useful in the treatment of septic wounds. In 1942, the compound hypericin was isolated from the leaves and flowers of St. John's wort and was found to be an effective sedative and restorative tonic for the nervous system. Today it is widely used as an anti-depressant, an anxiety reducer, and a treatment for chronic fatigue syndrome. As a blood purifier and cleanser, it has also been incorporated into leukemia treatments by homeopathic practitioners. Studies conducted by New York University researchers in 1988 concluded that St. John's wort controls the spread of viral infections, prevents tumor growth, and may be useful in combating the HIV virus. Results of those studies are still pending.

St. John's wort is most commonly found in capsule or tablet form and has one primary side effect—skin photosensitivity. Those taking this herb are advised to avoid exposure to strong sunlight.

Wheatgrass *(Poaceae spp.)*

Wheatgrass chlorophyll, contained in the first five to seven inches of the tender blades, is generally used to cleanse and purify bodily systems. It cleanses the colon, expels metals from the body, curtails development of bacteria, and stabilizes red blood cell counts. Bodybuilders often drink wheatgrass juice to increase and sustain energy and strength. Tagged a "chlorophyll super food," wheatgrass is now used for treating cancerous growths and other degenerative diseases. New studies have connected drinking wheatgrass juice with faster recovery rates from colon cancer.

Appendix 2

The Brain Game: Exercise to Train the Brain

Like all muscles in the body, the brain must be kept in shape to function at its optimum. Indeed, the adage "Use it or lose it" is most appropriate in reference to our higher intellectual powers! Taking ginkgo biloba, eating a healthy diet, and getting plenty of exercise will certainly help, but you also want to keep your brain active by continuing to learn and develop new interests throughout your life. In addition, if you perform simple exercises on a regular basis, you can "train your brain" to operate at peak levels of performance. The exercises below are mini-"workouts" for the brain, aimed at boosting the memory, increasing powers of concentration, and strengthening problem-solving capabilities.

MIND CALMERS

Workout #1: *Concentrate! How to clear and focus the mind*

The first step in any brain-training regime must involve a mental warm-up period. You must calm and quiet the clutter of your mind, pulling it into focus in order to achieve total concentration and build brainpower. To do this takes only 10 minutes a day, but you should perform it daily in order to develop high levels of concentration.

Begin by choosing a comfortable location and sit upright with your legs folded in front of you. Relax your body with deep inhalations (through the nose) and slow exhalations, thinking only of the process of air exchange breathing life into your body and brain. Pick up a familiar, simple object, an orange perhaps. Feel it: How does its skin feel on your fingertips? Smell it: Does it bring back any memories? What images does it conjure up? Imagine becoming smaller and smaller, so tiny that you could crawl inside that orange. Walk around it. How does it feel? What does it look like inside? How juicy or bright is it around you? Imagine leaving the orange and imagine yourself growing back to normal size while recalling all that you experienced, saw, felt, and tasted. Slowly count to five and you will feel awake and refreshed. Now your brain can focus on the tasks of the day.

Workout #2: *Improving your visual memory and concentration*

Repeat the exercise above with objects in your room—a chair, a tapestry, a lamp. Study the objects, feel and smell them, notice as much detail as possible. Now pretend that you are a camera, your eye the lens. Take some mental pictures. Find an open space on a wall and project those photos (with eyes open) onto the wall. Start with one photo at a time.

If you can't "develop" the "photo" fully, look back at the object and repeat the process until you can reproduce that object as an image on the wall. Do this until your mind's eye can see the image on the wall as clearly as your eyes saw the object itself. Over the period of a couple of weeks, increase the number of images you can project to build your powers of observation and recall. The more precisely your brain can code information, the better your powers of recall become. While the brain can store immense quantities of data, it does little for us if we can't retrieve the information when needed.

MIND EXPANDERS

Workout #3: *How to read faster and absorb more information*

By boosting your ability to read and comprehend, you can increase your power to learn. Simply paying attention to how fast you can read can significantly speed up your reading process without sacrificing comprehension. Next time you sit down to read a newspaper article or a chapter in a book, mark the point halfway through the piece you will read. Now read, noting the time you begin. Once you get to the halfway mark, stop and note the time again. How long did it take you?

Continue reading and concentrate on forcing yourself to read faster, but not so fast that you lose track of meaning. When you reach the end, note the time again.

Notice how much more quickly you read the second half. Just increasing your speed a bit more each time you read over a period of a few days or even weeks will provide noticeable results.

Workout #4: *Reading without repeating*

This exercise is the second stage of the one above. Even faster reading can be achieved by eliminating the tendency to "subvocalize"—repeating the words in your head as you read them.

Do you do this? Were you even aware of it? Often we do not trust our brain to absorb what has been read if we don't repeat the words as we read them, as if to "confirm" they've been read. Try reading a short piece without repeating. If it feels unnatural or difficult, try to increase your reading pace to a rate faster than you can repeat the words. It may feel like you do not know what you have read, but take a moment to jot down the key points of what you have read and you may be surprised at how much you did retain. Trust the brain and practice this until subvocalizing disappears.

MEMORY BOOSTERS

Workout #5: *How to remember lists*

Do you write lists—and then forget where you put them? Do you make a grocery list and then forget to bring it to the supermarket? Wouldn't it just be easier to remember what's on the list? This technique is short, simple, imaginative and fun. It can be used for long or short lists, and can easily be adapted to commit many types of lists to memory. It involves taking a "memory trip," combining the narrative flow of a story with the visualization of images quite familiar to you.

Prepare a route in your mind, one you now perform daily or perhaps one you remember vividly as a child—perhaps the road to Grandma's or the way to the supermarket. Choose recognizable landmarks from that route. Write down as many as you have items on your list to remember. For example, if my grocery list consists of turkey, cat food, potatoes, toilet paper, fingernail polish remover, and coffee, then I will pick six designated spots of my route to the supermarket: the front door, the tree in my front yard, the car, the stop sign at the end of my street, the ugly fuchsia house up the road, and the parking lot of the supermarket.

Next, picture taking this route and associate items on the list with your visual landmarks and create a story: I opened my *front door* and a *turkey* came rushing past me! It was chased up the *tree* by my *cat*, who was starving from lack of *food*. I finally made it to the *car*, which was filled with *potatoes* thanks to the neighborhood brats, who were also responsible for adorning the *stop sign* at the end of the road with *toilet paper*. However, much to my chagrin, that ugly house up the road finally had its fuchsia *paint removed*, but by the time I got to the supermarket the *parking lot* was flooded with *coffee*.

The designated landmarks of the route can remain the same, and the list changed to an order of events, a list of names or dates, or even a sequence of numbers. For example, to remember Mom's new phone number at work—627–1297—I may employ a rhyming technique to the order of landmarks: my front door *sticks*, a *shoe* tree, my cat with angel wings flying to *heaven*, and so on. Once this method is applied to short number sequences, it takes very little time before it is committed to memory.

Workout #6: *Remembering how to spell words correctly*

While the best way to improve your spelling is to read as much and as often as you can, it is quite easy to remind the mind of the correct spelling of words. Common spelling mistakes become habitual; once you misspell a word one time, you often misspell it all the time. The best way is to pull out a recent writing sample—a letter written to a friend, the first draft of a school paper. If you can't find one quickly, write a short piece of fiction or a fake letter to the editor of your newspaper. Have a friend proofread it, or run it through the spellcheck program on your computer.

Make a list of the misspelled words and look them up in the dictionary. Note the words' roots and syllable breaks, and find out the derivatives of the words. Then go over your list. Make the mistakes obvious to the brain—write and/or type the correct spelling numerous times, highlighting the forgotten letter or part of the word misspelled: nuge becomes nuDge, sevral becomes sevERal, concious conScious, and exercize ex-ER-ciSe. Break up the word, rearrange the syllables to emphasize the correct spelling (wed-NES-day), and see, in your mind's eye, the transformation of the word from wrong to right. Do this each time you finish writing and soon enough you will habitually spell well.

PROBLEM SOLVERS

Workout #7: *Making Decisions Decisively*

Do you have a decision to make but you just can't seem to come to a conclusion? Complicated decisions overload the mind with "ifs" and "buts" and mixed emotions. The familiar pros and cons list is an age-old technique that has survived because it works. But why not put a new spin on it?

When faced with a complicated decision, draw up a list of reasons for (pros) and reasons against (cons) and add a numerical value to each. For pros assign a value of +1 to +10; for cons, −1 to −10. Example: Should I go to graduate school in Texas? The pros are: The University of Texas is very well known for my field of study (+9); it would be a new experience for me to live in the South (+3); and the tuition fits my budget (+9). The cons: I don't want to live so far from my family (−10); I would rather live in a city like New York (−4); and I hate the heat and sun (−2).

Pros added up equal +21. Cons equal −16. Since the total figure adds up to +4, there is more chance that going to Texas may be the better option. The more positive or negative the total is, the clearer the decision. This method accounts for everything from major factors and trivial decisions to concrete logic and emotional bias.

Workout #8: *Perspectives on problem solving*

Sometimes when you don't have the solution to a problem, all you need is a bit of perspective. And sometimes when you gain perspective you find that you had the solution deep in your mind all along. This exercise is a creative approach to seeing a problem from many angles and from different points of view. It is a creative and far more effective spin on a "what would Mom do?" approach. Its purpose is to tap into more subconscious ideas, ideas you deny because of fear or insecurity, options that seem to you implausible, possibilities you didn't think were possible, solutions you thought not to exist.

Begin in a relaxed state; try this technique when you first wake up, when the mind is not yet cluttered with thoughts, worries, and lists of things to do. While lying in bed, breathe deeply and imagine your body becoming very light, so light that you begin to float above the bed, above the house and the city below. Float yourself to a forest. In this location you are to meet with five advisers—who will they be? Friends? Co-workers? Family? Historical figures or great leaders? Pick five people who you will explain your problem to. Meet with one at a time. What will you ask them? What will they ask you? Imagine, based on what you know about their personalities and achievements, how they will advise you. Do you agree or disagree with them? Tell them why. Let them respond.

Now move yourself to another clearing in the forest and meet with your next adviser. Discuss your options with him. What does he say? Once you have met with all of your advisers, return to your body, house, and bed. Slowly count to five while deep breathing, then write down any answers or options received during your "trip." You might be surprised to find what was inside of you all along and learn to trust in your own ability to see and think in perspective.

Glossary

Adrenal glands: Organs that sit atop each kidney and produce a variety of hormones, including the sex hormones (testosterone, estrogen, and progesterone), stress hormones (epinephrine and norepinephrine), and steroid hormones.

Aerobic exercise: Physical exercise that relies on oxygen for energy production.

Age-related macular degeneration: A vision disorder in which the macula becomes damaged as the tissue ages, causing difficulty reading and doing up-close work.

Allergens: Substances that cause manifestations of allergy; also called antigens.

Allergy: A disorder in which the body becomes hypersensitive to particular substances that provoke allergy symptoms through the release of certain immune system cells.

Alzheimer's disease: Brain disease associated with diffuse degeneration of brain cells, occurring mostly in old age.

Amino acids: Building blocks of protein molecules necessary for every bodily process.

Amygdala: A portion of the brain believed to be involved in mood, feeling, instinct, and possibly memory for recent events.

Anaerobic exercise: Exercise, including weight lifting
and isometrics, that draws upon the muscles for
stores of energy and does not require oxygen.

Angina pectoris: A disease of the heart involving severe
pain and a feeling of pressure in the chest, sometimes
radiating to the left shoulder and arm.

Angiogram: A diagnostic X ray of blood vessels or
other parts of the circulatory system.

Angioplasty: A surgical procedure altering the structure
of a heart vessel or using a balloon to expand or
remove blockage from the vessel.

Antibiotics: Any of a variety of natural or synthetic substances that inhibit the growth of or destroy bacteria.

Antibodies: Protein substances produced by immune
system cells that interact with and destroy cells or
microbes perceived to be foreign to the body.

Antigens: Substances foreign or perceived to be foreign
in the body, the presence of which result in the production of antibodies.

Antihistamines: Drugs that are often used to relieve
cold or allergy symptoms (i.e., Benadryl).

Anti-inflammatory: Substance, natural or pharmaceutical, that reduces swelling, inflammation, and pain.
Some common anti-inflammatory drugs are Feldene
(piroxicam), Motrin (ibuprofen), and Voltaren
(diclofenac sodium).

Antioxidant: Chemical molecule that prevents oxygen
from reacting with other compounds to create free
radicals. They protect cells from being damaged.

Arteries: Blood vessels that carry oxygenated blood

away from the heart to nourish cells throughout the body.

Arteriosclerosis: Disease involving thickening, hardening, and/or loss of elasticity in the artery walls, resulting in diminished function of tissues and organs. Used interchangeably with the term "atherosclerosis."

Aspirin: Drug that reduces inflammation and fever. Also known to affect the platelets to prevent thickening or clotting. Chemical name: acetylsalicyclic acid.

Autoimmune disease: Disease in which the immune system produces antibodies against the body's own cells, destroying healthy tissue.

Autonomic nervous system: The part of the nervous system primarily responsible for functions such as the heartbeat, blood pressure, and digestion. It is divided into two divisions, the sympathetic and the parasympathetic nervous system.

Axon: A nerve fiber that extends from the cell body of a neuron and carries nerve impulses away from it.

Beta amyloid plaques: The plaques that form within the brains of Alzheimer's disease patients that scientists believe are part of the disease process.

Biofeedback: A behavior-modification therapy in which people are taught to control bodily functions such as blood pressure through conscious effort.

Blood pressure: The force of blood on the walls of the arteries. Two types are measured: the higher, or systolic, pressure occurs each time the heart pushes blood into the vessels; the lower, or diastolic, pressure occurs when the heart is at rest.

Bronchioles: Subdivisions of the bronchial tubes.

Bronchodilators: Chemicals that relax or open the air passages in the lungs.

Bypass surgery: Surgical procedure used to create an

alternate route for blood to pass an obstruction, especially in the coronary arteries leading to and from the heart.

Capillaries: Any of the minute blood vessels, average 0.008 millimeters in diameter, carrying blood and forming the capillary system.

Carbohydrates: Organic compounds of carbon, hydrogen, and oxygen that include starches, cellulose, and sugars and are an important source of energy. Once consumed, all carbohydrates eventually break down into sugars.

Cardiac arrhythmia: Irregular beating of the heart.

Cardiovascular system: The heart together with the two networks of vessels: veins and arteries. Transports nutrients and oxygen to the tissues and removes waste products.

Cell membrane: Membrane that encloses the cell and is composed of proteins, lipids, and carbohydrates.

Central nervous system: The brain and spinal cord, which are responsible for the integration and production of all neurological functions.

Chinese medicine: A philosophy and methodology of health and medicine developed in ancient China.

Cholesterol: A fatlike substance found in the brain, nerves, liver, blood, and bile. Synthesized in the liver, cholesterol is essential in a number of bodily functions. In its oxidized—or bad—form, cholesterol contributes to the development of arteriosclerosis and other forms of cardiovascular disease.

Chronic: A disease or illness of long duration showing little change or of slow progression.

Coagulation: The process by which liquid blood changes to a jellylike mass, thereby stopping bleeding.

Conjuctiva: The mucous membrane that lines the eye and eyelid.

Corpora cavernosa: The pair of cylindrical blood sinuses that form the erectile tissue.

Coronary artery disease: A narrowing of the coronary arteries that prevents adequate blood supply to the heart muscle. Narrowing is usually caused by arteriosclerosis, and may progress to the point where the heart muscle is damaged.

Corticosteriods: Hormones produced in the cortex of the adrenal glands; drug versions of these hormones are used to treat inflammation.

CT scan: A tomogram (X-ray image) reconstituted by a computer to depict bone and soft tissues in several plans.

Depression: A medical illness marked by feelings of sadness, despair, and hopelessness, along with a host of physical symptoms such as weight loss, change in sleeps patterns, and others.

Dermatitis: Inflammation of the skin with itching, redness, and rashes.

DHEA: A natural steroid hormone secreted by the adrenal glands. Currently investigated as a potential aging trigger.

Diabetes mellitus: A disease caused by the failure of body cells to use carbohydrates, usually due to a lack of insulin or a failure of the body to use insulin properly; a major risk factor for cardiovascular disease.

Diabetic retinopathy: Damage to the blood vessels of the eyes due to uncontrolled or poorly controlled diabetes. One of the prime causes of blindness in older adults.

Diuretic: Any substance—natural or pharmaceutical—that works to lower the volume of blood by promoting salt and water excretion by way of the urine.

Dopamine: Amino acid found in the adrenal gland.

Edema: Accumulation of fluid in the tissues; may or may not be visible, and can be caused by injury, physical disorder, or leakage of fluids from capillaries or veins.

Electrocardiography (ECG or EKG): Diagnostic procedure that uses ultrasound waves to visualize structures in the heart.

Embolism: Blockage of an artery by a cluster of material circulating in the bloodstream. The particle, called an embolus, can be a blood clot, an air bubble, bacteria, cholesterol, or any other substance.

Endocrine system: System of glands and other structures that secrete hormones into the bloodstream, including the adrenals, ovaries, pancreas, pineal, pituitary, testes, and thyroid.

Endorphins: Natural substances produced by the body that function as natural painkillers.

Epinephrine: Hormone secreted by the adrenal glands that increases heart rate and constricts blood vessels.

Erectile dysfunction: Also called impotence; the inability to attain or maintain an erection.

Essential fatty acids: Unsaturated fatty acids that cannot be synthesized in the body and are considered essential for maintaining health. Some types of fish contain high levels of essential fatty acids.

Estrogen: A group of female hormones responsible for the development of secondary sex traits and aspects of reproduction. Produced in the ovaries, adrenal glands, and fatty tissue.

Fat: The principal form in which energy is stored in the body.

Fight-or-flight response: The body's response to perceived danger or stress, involving the release of hormones and subsequent rise in heart rate, blood pressure, and muscle tension.

Free radicals: Molecules containing an odd number of electrons, making it highly reactive and, as a result, potentially dangerous to healthy cells.

Gangrene: Death of tissue, usually due to loss of the blood supply.

Ginkgo biloba: A deciduous tree that provides the leaves from which a medicinal extract is derived.

Flavonoids: A group of substances found in many plants and fruits that act as antioxidants.

Flavona glycosides: The antioxidant components of ginkgo biloba, including quercetin, kaempferol, and isorhamnetin.

Glaucoma: Eye disease in which loss of vision occurs because of an abnormally high pressure in the eye.

Glucose: The most common simple sugar; an essential source of energy for the body.

Heart attack: Also called myocardial infarction. Death of heart tissue caused by an interruption of blood circulation through the coronary arteries.

Heart rate: The number of times the heart beats (contracts and releases) each minute.

Hemoglobin: The component in red blood cells responsible for carrying oxygen through the bloodstream to cells of the body.

High-density lipoprotein (HDL): A lipid-carrying protein that transports the so-called "good" cholesterol away from the artery walls to the liver for excretion.

Histamine: A compound related to the allergic response; causes dilation of blood vessels and contraction of smooth muscle and is an important mediator of inflammation.

Holistic: Pertaining to the whole body; holistic treatment of disease considers every part of the body as it works to bring the internal environment into balance.

Hormone: Chemical produced by the endocrine system that, when secreted, has a specific effect on other organs and processes. Hormones are often referred to as "chemical messengers," and they influence such diverse activities as growth, sexual development, metabolism, and sleep cycles. Hormones are also instrumental in maintaining the proper internal chemical and fluid balance.

Hypothalamus: Portion of the brain that activates, controls, and integrates part of the nervous system, endocrine processes, and many bodily functions, such as temperature, sleep, and appetite.

Immunity: The quality of being highly resistant to a disease or antigen after initial exposure and response by the immune system.

Immunoglobulin: One of a group of structurally related proteins that act as antibodies.

Infarction: The death of tissue that occurs when the blood supply to a localized part of the body is blocked.

Inflammation: A normal immune response to injury or infection. Chronic inflammation results in redness, heat, swelling, pain, and loss of function in the affected area.

Insomnia: A chronic inability to go to sleep or remain asleep. Caused by a variety of factors, including diet and exercise habits, emotional stress, and hormonal imbalances.

Insulin: The hormone, secreted by the pancreas, responsible for the use of glucose as energy by body cells.

Ischemia: Oxygen deficiency caused by an obstruction of a blood vessel.

Leukocyte: A type of white blood cell involved in the immune response.

Limbic system: A group of brain structures that influence the endocrine and autonomic motor systems; thought to be the seat of emotions.

Lipids: Fats, steroids, phospholipids, and glycolipids; fat or fatlike substances.

Low-density lipoprotein (LDL): A protein composed of fats, large amounts of cholesterol, and triglycerides. LDL is the "bad" cholesterol considered a risk factor for cardiovascular disease.

Melatonin: Hormone released into the bloodstream by the pineal gland. Melatonin production is stimulated by darkness and inhibited by light and is known to act as a sleep promoter, antioxidant, and immune system booster.

Meridians: In traditional Chinese medicine, the channels in the body through which *qi* runs.

Nicotine: A chemical substance derived from tobacco that affects blood pressure and heart rate.

Neurotransmitters: Substances that transmit messages to, from, and within the brain and other tissues. Serotonin, norepinephrine, acetylcholine, and dopamine are among the many neurotransmitters that send and receive messages in the brain and body.

Norepinephrine: Hormone secreted by the adrenal gland as a reaction to the "fight-or-flight" response that raises blood pressure and acts to stimulate muscle contraction.

Obesity: Usually considered to be present when a person is 20 percent above the recommended weight for his or her body.

Parasympathetic nervous system: The division of the nervous system that, when stimulated, slows heart rate, lowers blood pressure, and slows respiration.

Pathogens: Disease-causing organisms.

Peripheral vascular disease: Cardiovascular disease that affects the outlying blood vessels, such as those in the legs.

Phytochemicals: Beneficial substances found in plant material and used as medicine.

Pineal gland: Endocrine gland located in the brain that secretes the hormone melatonin. The pineal gland begins to shrink and calcify during the aging process, thereby significantly reducing the amount of circulating melatonin.

Placebo: A medicine that is ineffective but may help to relieve a condition because the patient has faith in its powers.

Plaque: Fatty deposits that build up on the inner walls of the blood vessels, resulting in obstruction of the normal flow of blood.

Platelet: A disk-shaped substance in the blood primarily responsible for blood clotting.

Platelet-activating factor (PAF): A substance produced during the inflammatory response that triggers the platelets to coagulate, or form clots. It is also associated with inflammation in the skin and the bronchi.

Premenstrual syndrome: Constellation of physical and emotional symptoms related to hormonal changes associated with the second half of the menstrual cycle.

Qi: In traditional Chinese medicine, the life force or energy of the body and the universe.

Raynaud's disease: A condition in which exposure to cold temperatures causes the blood vessels of the fingers and toes to constrict, cutting off the blood supply.

Retina: A light-sensitive layer of nerve cells that lines the back of the eye and converts light to nerve impulses, resulting in sight.

Retinopathy: Damage to the retina, a common complication of diabetes. It occurs when the small blood vessels become larger and leak fluid into the center of the retina.

Risk factor: Condition or behavior that increases one's likelihood of developing a disease or injury.

Sclerosis: An abnormal thickening or hardening of the arteries and veins.

Serotonin: A naturally occurring neurotransmitter derived from the amino acid tryptophan.

Stress: Any factor, physical or emotional, that requires a response or change. Excess or chronic stress threatens the health of the body.

Stroke: An interruption of the blood flow to the brain, causing damage and loss of function.

Sympathetic nervous system: Division of the autonomic nervous system responsible for such actions as blood pressure, salivation, and digestion; works in balance with the parasympathetic nervous system.

Symptoms: Observable or internal changes in the mental, emotional, and physical condition.

Synapse: The tiny gap across which nerve impulses pass from one neuron to the next.

Terpene lactones: The substances in ginkgo biloba that help prevent blood from clotting. They include the bilobalides and ginkgolides A, B, C, and J.

Testosterone: The primary male sex hormone responsible for male sex characteristics.

Thrombosis: The formation of a blood clot, called a thrombus, that partially or completely blocks a blood vessel.

Tincture: An alcoholic solution of a medicinal substance.

Tinnitus: A condition characterized by ringing, roaring, hissing, and/or buzzing noises in the ears; usually of unknown origin.

Transient ischemic attack: An interruption of blood supply to a part of the brain that causes temporary impairment of vision, speech, or movement; can be a warning sign of stroke.

Triglyceride: The most common lipid found in fatty tissue; the form in which fat is stored in the body.

Vascular: Pertaining to or supplied with blood vessels.

Yin-Yang: Chinese concept that describes all existence in terms of states or conditions that are different but mutually dependent; traditional Chinese medicine aims to restore balance to these contrasting aspects of the body and mind.

Resources

Negotiating your way through health care options—natural and mainstream—is a daunting enterprise, especially today when so many doors to new treatments and approaches are now open. Following is a list of associations and organizations that provide products and/or more information about ginkgo biloba and other subjects you've read about in this book. In addition, we provide a brief bibliography of some of the new and older books you can read to find out more about alternative medicine. Remember: Knowledge *is* power. Take advantage of these resources if you're interested in improving your general health.

Ginkgo Biloba Extract

Below are some suppliers and companies known for producing and selling high-quality products:

American WholeHealth, Inc.
(800) 841–5523
(781) 641–3480 (fax)

American WholeHealth Centers offer physician-supervised alternative medicine, combining high medical standards with a caring philosophy and practice. They have a fully stocked natural medicine apothecary, with high-quality GBE in capsule and tincture form. Call or fax and request a catalog. Mail order is readily available, and there is an automatic shipping policy.

Two major companies known to produce good-quality herbal remedies are PhytoPharmica and Nature's Way. You can find their products in health food stores around the country.

Acupuncture/Chinese Medicine

American Holistic Medical Association
4101 Lake Boone Trail, Suite 201
Raleigh, NC 27607
(919) 787–5181

American Academy of Medical Acupuncture
5820 Wilshire Boulevard, Suite 500
Los Angeles, CA 90036
(213) 937–5514

Qi-Gong Institute/East-West Academy of Healing Arts
450 Sutter Street
San Francisco, CA 94108
(415) 788–2227

Allergies

American Academy of Environmental Medicine
P.O. Box 16106
Denver, CO 80216
(303) 622–9755

Asthma and Allergy Foundation of America
1124 15th Street, N.W.
Washington, DC 20005
(202) 466–7643
800-7-ASTHMA

Alzheimer's Disease

Alzheimer's Disease and Related Disorders
919 North Michigan Avenue, Suite 1000
Chicago, IL 60611
(800) 272–3900
On-line contact: http://www.alz.org

Biofeedback

Association for Applied Psychophysiology and Biofeedback
10200 West 44th Avenue, Suite 304
Wheat Ridge, CO 80033
(303) 422–8436

Center for Applied Psychophysiology
Menninger Clinic
P.O. Box 829
Topeka, KS 66601
(913) 273–7500

Depression

American Psychological Association
750 First Street, N.E.
Washington, DC 20002
(202) 336–5500

Depression Awareness, Recognition, and Treatment (D/ART)
Program Department GL
Room 10–855600 Fishers Lane
Rockville, MD 20857
(800) 421–4211

Healthy Aging

American Association for Retired People
601 E Street, N.W.
Washington, DC 20049
(202) 434–2277
On-line contact: http://www.aarp.org

Herbal Medicine

The American Botanical Council
P.O. Box 201660
Austin, TX 78720
(512) 331–8868

Herb Research Foundation
1007 Pearl Street, Suite 200
Boulder, CO 80302
(303) 449–2265

The Herb Quarterly
Long Mountain Press
P.O. Box 689
San Anselmo, CA 94960
(415) 455–9540

Eclectic Institute
4385 Southeast Lusted Road
Sandy, OR 97055
(800) 332–4372

Impotence

The Gedding Obson Sr. Foundation
Impotence Resource Center
(800) 433–4211
On-line contact: http://www.impotence.org

Meditation and Mind/Body Medicine

The Center for Mind-Body Studies
5225 Connecticut Avenue, N.W.
Washington, DC 20015
(202) 966–7388

Stress Reduction Clinic
University of Massachusetts Medical Center
55 Lake Avenue North
Worcester, MA 01655

Nutrition

Center for Science in the Public Interest
1875 Connecticut Avenue, N.W.
Washington, DC 20009
(202) 332–9110
On-line contact: http://www.cspinet.org

Yoga

Himalayan Institute of Yoga, Science, and Philosophy
RRI Box 400
Honesdale, PA 18431
(800) 822–4547

International Association of Yoga Therapists
109 Hillside Avenue
Mill Valley, CA 94941
(415) 383–4587

Reading List

Beinfeld, Harriet, and Efrem Korngold. *Between Heaven and Earth: A Guide to Chinese Medicine.* New York: Ballantine, 1991.

Benson, Herbert. *The Relaxation Response.* New York: Outlet Books, Inc. 1993.

Berg, Robert L., and Joseph S. Cassels, eds. *The Second Fifty Years: Promoting Health and Preventing Disability.* Institute of Medicine. Washington, D.C.: National Academy Press, 1990.

Borysenko, Joan. *Fire in the Soul.* New York: Warner Books, 1994.

Castleman, Michael. *Natural Cures*. Emmaus, PA: Rodale Press, 1995.

Collins, James F. *Your Eyes: An Owner's Guide*. New York: Prentice Hall, 1995.

Dossey, Larry. *Healing Words: The Power of Prayer and the Practice of Medicine*. New York: Harper, 1995.

Futterman, Lori. *The PMS and Perimenopausal Sourcebook*. Los Angeles: Lowell House, 1997.

Gladstar, Rosemary. *Herbal Healing for Women*. New York: Fireside, 1993.

Greer, Rita. *Antioxidant Nutrition*. New York: Souvenir Press, 1996.

Halpern, Georges, M.D. *Ginkgo: A Practical Guide*. Garden City Park, NY: Avery, 1998.

Hobbs, Christopher. *Ginkgo: Elixir of Youth*. Loveland, CO: Interweave Press, 1991.

Hoffman, David. *The New Holistic Herbal*. San Francisco: Element, 1991.

Kaptchuk, Ted. *The Web That Has No Weaver*. New York: Congdon and Weed, 1992.

Kirschmann, Gayla. *Nutrition Almanac*. New York: McGraw-Hill, 1996.

Lad, Vasant. *The Yoga of Herbs*. San Francisco: Lotus Lights, 1986.

LeVert, Suzanne. *Melatonin: The Anti-Aging Hormone*. New York: Avon, 1995.

Mathiasen, Patrick, and Suzanne LeVert. *Late Life Depression*. New York: Dell, 1997.

McClain, Gary, Ph.D. *The Natural Way of Healing Asthma and Allergies*. New York: Dell, 1995.

Moyers, Bill. *Healing and the Mind*. New York: Doubleday, 1993.

Murray, Michael T. *Male Sexual Vitality*. Rocklin, CA: Prima Publishing, 1994.

Randolph, Theron, M.D. *An Alternative Approach to Allergies*. New York: HarperPerennial, 1990.

Reid, Daniel. *The Complete Book of Chinese Health and Healing*. Boston: Shambala, 1994.

Rothfeld, Glenn, and Suzanne LeVert. *Natural Medicine for Allergies*. Emmaus, PA: Rodale Press, 1997.

Teeguardan, Ron. *Chinese Tonic Herbs*. Los Angeles: Japan Publications, 1987.

Tierra, Lesley. *The Herbs of Life*. New York: Crossing Press, 1992.